I0776779

Dealing With Life's Changes

As Time Goes By

EVA BENNETT

BALBOA.PRESS

A DIVISION OF HAY HOUSE

Balboa Press books may be ordered through booksellers or by contacting:

Balboa Press
A Division of Hay House
1663 Liberty Drive
Bloomington, IN 47403
www.balboapress.com.au
AU TFN: 1 800 844 925 (Toll Free inside Australia)
AU Local: 0283 107 086 (+61 2 8310 7086 from outside Australia)

Also by Eva Bennet
"So What Do We Do Now?" The Baby Boomers' Guide to Enjoying Retirement

Print information available on the last page.

ISBN: 978-1-9822-9093-1 (sc)
ISBN: 978-1-9822-9094-8 (e)

Balboa Press rev. date: 06/26/2021

TESTIMONIALS

"Your book is a very enlightening look into the types of issues, people dealing with change have to face. I love your use of real-life examples and also the quotes you have used which re-enforce the messages you are promoting.

I spend my working life educating others and assisting them to manage their financial affairs. It has been very fulfilling to see a gradual shift in the trend, of Australians taking greater control of their own financial future in recent times. However in saying that, it pains me to see these same Australians neglecting their personal health and well-being in the process.

It is so refreshing to see Eva provide real life examples in her books and at seminars, to assist people with managing the non-financial stresses of life, by providing a great recipe of tips to combat these stresses head on. She has reminded me also, to stay positive and focus on the important things in life. I hope you truly enjoy this honest account from Eva in her new book, "As Time Goes By" and that it provides you with the skills and mindset, to make the most of the life that is still ahead of you." - C.Wood, Operations Manager, ACSRF Sydney NSW

"Congratulations on your new book. You have made it easy to read and covered so many important topics with great insight and clarity which people can relate to, whatever stage of life they are at. Eva's book takes you on a journey, which many people have not thought about, but can associate with. The reader is given direction on how they can work through their issues, to create their own resolution, which is important.

For a number of years now, I have had the pleasure of speaking alongside Eva, at a number of client seminars, covering a range of topics people should consider as they enter retirement. Eva has thought through so many of the topics that confront retirees and she provides solutions on how to deal with them. Whether it's listening to Eva speak on this subject or reading her book, she provides help, understanding and guidance, on how the audience or reader, can resolve these issues and pave the way for a wonderful retirement." – C. Martin, Business Development Manager, AMP –Brisbane Qld

"After the events that have changed my life during the last few years, reading this book has reassured me, that our positivity and thoughts can really help us in how we approach and deal with the many different situations in our daily lives. A truly interesting and thought provoking book, that is easy to read and can be enjoyed by all." – C. French, teacher NSW.

CONTENTS

COVID -19 Pandemic Dealing With Life's Changes...............ix

Introduction...xi

Chapter 1   The 3 R's –...1

Chapter 2   Catch Your Thoughts - Change Your
             Thoughts - Change Your Life 5

Chapter 3   Endings and New Beginnings 15

Chapter 4   Take The Plunge 21

Chapter 5   Ask and You Will Receive................................26

Chapter 6   Breath of Calm 31

Chapter 7   The Changing Face of Retirement 35

Chapter 8   Re-invent Yourself 40

Chapter 9   Service to Others...45

Chapter 10   "Till Death Us Do Part."................................50

Chapter 11   Communicating with Others 59

Chapter 12   Are You Connected or Disconnected?...............67

Chapter 13   The Financial Diet...71

Chapter 14   Life is a Balancing Act 80

Chapter 15   Lighten The Load..86

Chapter 16   Pull All The Weeds Out Now!.........................90

Chapter 17   Slow Down the Ageing Process.........................92

Chapter 18   Looking Younger Naturally..............................99

Chapter 19   The 6 Ingredients to Cook Up A Great Life.....106

Remember to....... 111

COVID -19 PANDEMIC
DEALING WITH LIFE'S CHANGES

Just recently, I had a 'light bulb ' moment, that the book I wrote 8 years ago, "As Time Goes By, Dealing With Life's Changes" is perfect for helping people to deal with this incredible year of the COVID-19 Pandemic.

Many of the chapters in this book, explore the ways in which we can all deal with the different kinds of major changes that can happen in our lives. Be it your health — mental, emotional, physical or social, relationships or finances, to name a few, my suggestions have helped many people resolve issues and improve the quality oftheir lives — to live a healthier, happier life & slow down the ageing process.

Every chapter gives tips on how to deal with all of issues. An important one is about how we think. Research shows that our mental health has a big impact on our emotions & physical health.. My motto is:- Catch your thoughts — Change your thoughts — Change your life. Very powerful!

Another important issue is how to communicate more effectively in any kind of relationship. My chapter on communicating effectively, gives easy to follow tips on how to do this.

Since early this year, when COVID took hold, there has been a sharp rise in mental health issues & suicide. I see my book & the stories from people that are in my book, that each small step you take to live a more positive life, helps you to come to terms with the unexpected changes that come into our lives.

So many people over the last 8 years, have let me know how my book has helped them to resolve issues and pave the way for a better quality of life which is wonderful.

I truly believe that if you read my book, which many people have said is easy to read, and practise the suggestions I have made & used myself, you will be able to change your life for the better.

Eva Bennett

INTRODUCTION

"As Time Goes By" has been created around a collection of articles I have written as time has gone by. Using the knowledge and experiences that I have gained over the past 25 years, running numerous seminars and personal development programs, I want to share with you, practical suggestions that can work and bring positive changes into your life.

The theme of my book is on how to handle changes in our lives. Besides dealing with major changes like retirement, redundancy and relationships, the suggestions I discuss are also relevant for other changes that can affect our life like ageing, moving, illness, financial loss, natural disasters. I think you'll be surprised how most of the chapters will be relevant to you in some way, no matter what age group you are. The topics I cover and the special stories that other people have kindly allowed me to share, will give you insights and suggestions on how to handle change on different levels, so that you can make the most of your life on this earth.

I strongly believe, that the main underlying 'ingredient' that influences how we deal with all aspects of our life, is **how we think** and this affects how we do handle change.

It is my wish that the chapters in this book inspire you, but don't overwhelm you with too much information too soon, so that you can confidently start making the changes in your life that are relevant to your needs. *"A journey of a thousand miles begins with one step."* Lao Tzu.

Instead of trying to make too many changes at once and finding it all too hard, begin with one thing you can change. When that has been successful, gradually step-by-step, make other changes to improve your life.

> Confucius said: *"I hear and I forget, I see and I remember, I do and I understand."*

I trust that you will enjoy reading my second book and look forward to your feedback.

Acknowledgements

Special thanks to the people who contributed their personal stories for publication and I respect their wish for me to only use their first names.

My heartfelt thanks to those who made time in their busy schedules, to proof-read my manuscript. I valued their support and feedback.

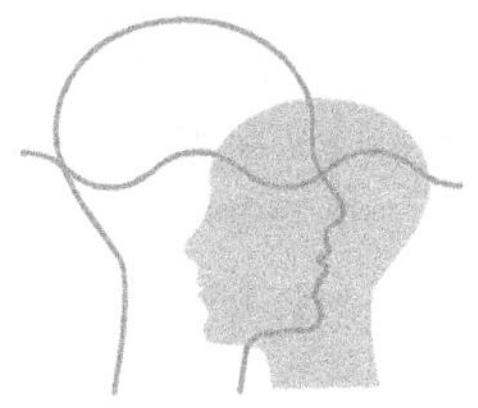

1

The 3 R's –

Reflection.....Resilience......Renewal

Reflection –*"What went wrong? Why is this happening to me? What have I done?"* Every so often we may experience an unexpected turn of events in our life. This can make us feel 'lost', directionless and disconnected. As *'dark'* as that period can seem, and I have been there, it is a natural process to go through, if we are to grow and move on. During this void, which can last from a few days to a few months depending on the situation, we need to reflect on what we have been doing and what we could do differently. Eventually we will see the light at the end of the tunnel and move on.

Rather than looking with regret at what we may not have done, we can now look at the new opportunities that are possible. In this reflection process, we can start a 'bucket list' of the things we would still like to do in our lives. This gives us something to look forward to.

Resilience – After the big changes that retirement, redundancy and relationships can bring into our lives, resilience helps us to 'bounce back'. No matter how well-prepared you think you are for a new beginning like retirement for example, many people can find that initially it can be a shock to the system, when the reality kicks in that you are not going back to your workplace. Anxiety can take hold, now that the familiar routines and structures are gone. If not dealt with, it can lead to depression, particularly for men. Staying positive, seeking help, overcoming fear thoughts and believing that you can move through this transition period is all part of being resilient. In the following chapters, you will learn more details about strategies to deal with endings.

<u>This is an inspiring story of resilience</u>: In 1972, a 40 year old man was injured in a bad car accident. Among other injuries, he had a damaged liver which was a serious problem. As he could not return to work, because of the extent of his injuries, he said to the doctor, *"What have I got to live for?"* The doctor replied, *"Look out the window and see the horizon. Start walking and keep walking towards it. Life is a journey."* Today that same man, now 80 years of age, is fit and walks daily. He developed a strong will to live.

Watching the telecast of the 2012 London Paralympic Games, was a wonderful example of the resilience of the disabled athletes, as they competed enthusiastically in the various events. I was in awe of their determination to live life to the full and not let their disabilities stop them.

Resilience in times of economic downturn is important as well - to keep moving on with life and believing that things can only get better. Research is finding that people who maintain an optimistic outlook, can live up to 12 years longer and in better health, than someone who has a pessimistic outlook.

Renewal – The time spent on reflection helps our outlook to be more hopeful and positive, Keeping our mental and physical health balanced, makes us more resilient. When we see that redundancy can lead to new opportunities, that new relationships are possible, and that retirement can be an exciting new beginning, we are not caught up in dwelling on the past. We bounce back with renewed energy, re-inventing ourselves and regaining the feeling of self-worth we had before. We explore the opportunities that are available in our community, to use our skills and talents to help others. We now have the time to learn new skills. Life takes on new meaning, we make new friends, we maintain our health and we can **enjoy life**!

There is a fourth **R** that we don't want to have, and that is **Regrets.**

The following list of regrets or disappointments of life, have been found to be common among older people as they approach the end of their lives.

- Not living out your dreams and desires.
- Not having any dreams to fulfil.
- Spending too much time working and not enough with your family and friends.
- Not knowing how to be truly happy.
- Trying too hard and spending too much time on things that in the big picture weren't important.
- Not taking care of your health.
- Not contributing to the community and making a difference.

Check if you may be heading towards any of the above, or have any of these regrets already. It's never too late to start addressing them now and take action to start changing. Much of what I have written about in this book, gives suggestions that can guide you.

We only have one life, so make the most of it, before it's too late.

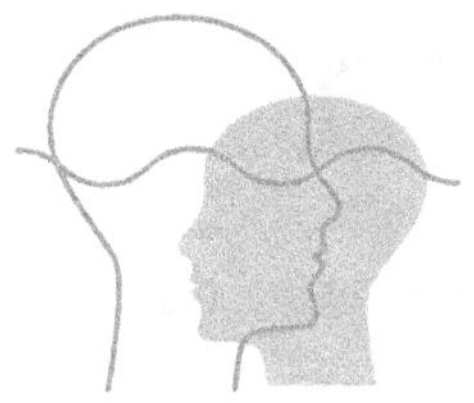

2

Catch Your Thoughts - Change Your Thoughts - Change Your Life

What are you thinking? How are you feeling? Did you know that over 60,000 thoughts run through our minds each day? Whether the majority of those thoughts are positive or whether they are negative, our thoughts influence our emotions and in turn our physical health. This was confirmed by scientific research carried out in the 1970's. Up till then, much of the medical fraternity did not believe this. The results of the research found that minute chemicals called neuro-peptides, acted as *'communicator molecules'* in our bodies, whereby the neurons of the brain can *'talk'* to the rest of the body.

A few years later it was found that neuro-peptides were in the immune system and other body organs like the heart and liver, as well. The chemicals in the brain form a continuous circuit not only with the receptors of the brain, but also with other body parts. This makes it physiologically impossible to separate the mind from the body. Professor Candance Pert says that *"Your mind is in every cell of your body."* So, if we focus constantly on fear thoughts, we are inviting ill-health into our lives.

I have a lovely friend who has rarely been sick in the 30 years that I have known her. When I went down to visit her last year, I was amazed at the sight of red scabs all over her arms and legs, which had literally appeared overnight a couple of weeks earlier. The doctor was treating her for **psoriasis**, a skin disease she has never had before in her life! As it turns out, she had recently had major dental surgery. I hadn't known that she had been petrified for the three months leading up to the surgery, as she is normally such a positive, cheerful person. As well as that, she had the added stress of having to prepare for a major house renovation.

So with all the stress going on in her life – the fear thoughts of facing the dental surgery and also the house renovation, her body re-acted and she developed psoriasis. Interestingly, in her book, *'You Can Heal Your Body'* Louise Hay says that the thought pattern that can cause psoriasis, is the **fear of being hurt**. My friend and I discussed the Body-Mind connection and how our repetitive thought patterns can either keep us healthy or can cause sickness.

As my friend still needed a further session of the dental surgery, which she was not looking forward to, I suggested that instead of staying focused on her fear of the dental surgery, she could turn her thoughts around to: *"I now feel calm about the dental surgery and trust that everything will go safely and smoothly and I will have beautiful teeth."* Every time she started to feel fearful, she could catch her thoughts and replace them with the above statement. This new thought pattern, repeated regularly, gradually calmed her fear and helped the psoriasis to heal.

Actually the belief that our thoughts create our reality has been around for a long time, as early as the bible. In 1925, Florence Shinn wrote a booklet called *"The Game of Life"* in which she shows how to use the power of your thoughts to become a winner in life. In 1937, Napoleon Hill wrote his famous book, *"Think and Grow Rich"* which is still read today. Once the body-mind connection was proven scientifically, many more people have taken that information on board.

Our thoughts are very powerful because they trigger the way we feel at any given moment. Our feelings then determine our actions and behaviour and leads to the results we experience in our daily lives – good or bad. If you constantly think negative thoughts, the subconscious mind will start to accept these thoughts and make them come true. For example, if you constantly think of getting poor customer service when you go shopping, that's what you are likely to get. If you think *"I get great customer service"* then that is what you are more likely to get. The words we use in our self-talk, can create our reality. How can we un-invite negative thought patterns? By catching your thoughts, you can change your thoughts and so change your life.

Your mind can only hold one thought
at a time, so make it a good one!

We **do** have the ability to change the way we think! Just as the AFL football player trains for hours to perfect kicking the ball off the right foot and then the left foot, until it becomes an automatic response, so can you also **re-train your brain** to think more positively and less negatively, until that becomes an automatic response. That is why some people handle adversity well, while others plummet into despair, because of their dominant thinking pattern.

Australian athlete, Sally Pearson won the **gold medal** at the 2012 London Olympics in the 100m hurdles. During the interview after the race, she spoke about how she kept telling herself before the start of the race, *"It is now my time to win."* She would have used the word *'win'* at least six times during the interview and never had a fear thought that she might not be able to do it. She added, that she showed her determination, by keeping her focus on being the winner, each time she crossed a hurdle. She won by 200th of a second. How is that for creating a positive mindset! Words are powerful and I think focusing on the word 'win' was more powerful than focusing on wanting the 'gold medal'.

The first step to increasing positive thoughts is to dissolve negative thoughts. Over the next few weeks, when a negative thought pops up, jot it down. What is causing this thought? Now re-frame that thought. For example: Instead of thinking, *"I am really nervous about speaking at the meeting."* Re-frame as: *"I now speak confidently at the meeting."* Each time you catch yourself sliding back to the fear thought, say the positive one to yourself. Like the AFL footballer perfecting his kick, it will take time, effort and persistence to change old thinking patterns. The more you use this technique, the less stress you will feel in your life.

Here is a simple exercise, that takes a few minutes each morning, to 'kick-start' your day in a positive way. This is a list that I use and re-write every so often. You can put one list on your bedroom wall and perhaps keep one at work or even in your bag, for when you need to re-charge the mind. I do this regularly, to keep myself from sliding into negative moods.

Today..............

- I am thankful for my good health.
- I remember to take slow, deep breaths during the day, especially when I feel stressed.
- I breathe in confidence and breathe out fear.
- I remember to drink water regularly.
- I go for a walk in the fresh air.
- I now keep an open mind about what happens in my life.
- I now see the glass half full instead of half empty.
- I am kind to myself.
- I see the best in others
- I am open to amazing and wonderful opportunities flowing into my life.

I find that creating a list of positive comments relevant to your life, can reduce the negative thought patterns and reduce the stress that can build up in your life. You can only have one thought at a time, so make it positive.

William James has this great quote – ***"The greatest discovery in my life is that a human being can alter his life by altering his attitude."***

I recently came across an article in the newspaper that stated – "Of almost 1,500 breast cancer survivors, whose views were collated for research, 23% blamed stress as having contributed to them getting cancer. Many studies have proven the **stress >< disease** connection. Feeling stressed develops from repetitive negative thoughts as I mentioned earlier. A Canadian researcher showed that heart disease patients who were given stress-reduction guidance and then monitored for stress levels, were half as likely to die from cardiac problems, compared to a similar group that was not given such help.

We all have ups and downs in our lives and we can easily slide into negative thinking. No one is saying that we must eliminate stress from our lives in order to be healthy, but we can try to manage and reduce it. Some stress is actually good for us. I like to use what I call the 80/20 rule. If we can spend 80% of our time thinking positively, we have a much better chance to live a healthier life, than if we spend 80% of our time thinking negatively.

Cheryl's Story – How My Life Changed.

"Over a number of years, my kidneys had been slowly deteriorating and no one in the medical world, could explain why. 90% of kidney problems can usually be identified. As my body was retaining fluid and my kidneys weren't able to rid my body of the various toxins, I had to start having dialysis in 2010 at the age of 53. I was doing home dialysis 3 days a week, each session lasting 5 hours, to keep my body functioning.

My life and also my partner's life changed because of the dialysis. Social activities and even my work as a teacher revolved around the dialysis sessions and also depended on how I was feeling. During this challenging time, I was fortunate to be surrounded by wonderful people —my partner, my family, the hospital staff at the home dialysis centre. These people helped me to realise the importance of being positive and accepting, that what I was going through wasn't the ideal situation, but it was for the benefit of my long term health. Also that I was fortunate to still be able to do things like going on walks, but I had to stop playing hockey, because it's a contact sport. Yes, there were many times that I wondered, if this was how the rest of my life was going to be. Would I ever be able to go on a holiday again? Would I have to forever organise my future weekly activities around dialysis sessions?

Then a year later, I received the gift of life – a kidney from my partner. Testing of my close family members had not been successful, so my partner had gone through 12 months of tests to see if his kidney was compatible and it was! For the next 5 months, my partner and I rented an apartment to be near the city hospital. Each day, I had to go to the hospital, to be attached to a dialysis machine for plasma treatment to cleanse the blood.

This is when I fully realised the importance of having a positive attitude and keeping the negative thoughts out of my mind. The wonderful nursing staff at the hospital helped me to realise, how to take just one day at a time and only deal with what was happening on that day. I learnt not to look too far ahead. It was also important to smile and be thankful. While staying in the city, I found that simple every day pleasures meant a lot. I would often talk to myself in my mind and tell myself that **"everything will be fine."** These conversations with myself were particularly important, whenever I began to feel a bit depressed.

Eventually I was well enough to go home. This was a great feeling. It became very apparent that I had made it through the past few months, not only because of my wonderful support team, but also because of the way I had approached the situation. If something wasn't going the way it was supposed to, instead of letting worrying thoughts take over, I would tell myself **"It will get better and tomorrow is another day."**

I have recently returned to primary teaching, but now in a part-time role. I've been teaching for 32 years and enjoy it. I was missing the regular interaction with my colleagues and students. Teaching keeps my mind occupied and the pay is handy. I must admit, it hasn't been an easy path, returning to the work force. I am having to really put into practise, what I have worked hard at over the past year and that is – **Be Positive and Be Happy!**

My kidney transplant is not a cure, but it is a 'holiday' from the dialysis machine – a very long holiday I hope! This experience has taught me a lot about myself. I was always a person who had to be organised and know exactly what was happening the following month. Now I live for each day. I find that I am more relaxed and I enjoy what is happening around me at that particular moment. I truly believe that I am a much happier person and I am able to control my thoughts and attitude. As a result of this stronger mind set, I deal better with whatever comes my way. I am definitely a healthier person because of this. When something negative begins to take over my thoughts, I stop and tell myself, "This is *not good for my well being or for my continued process to have a healthy and contented life." I am now probably the fittest and healthiest I have ever been.*

This is because of, not only the medication and a healthier lifestyle, but also realising what is important, such as finding the good things about each day and remembering to be happy. I also believe that, surrounding yourself with positive people impacts on the way you live your own life. P.S. I am still talking to myself each day!"

"Sound mind - Sound Body."

At various times we hear about people who have been involved in serious accidents and been told that they may never walk again. Some of those people take that statement as fact and never do walk again. Others are determined to prove that they will walk again and set themselves a goal to be up and walking by a certain time. Then they start doing whatever it takes, to bring this into reality. When you read their stories, they were determined to live the best life they could and focused on whatever they could do, to conquer their injury and have ended up amazing their doctors. Watching the telecast of the 2012 Paralympics in London, showed the amazing determination of those in the wheelchair events, and how having no legs was not going to stop them enjoying life.

As mentioned earlier, it is our mind-set, positive or negative, that creates our feelings, which then create our behaviour. The language that we use can reflect what we are thinking, as can the tone of our voice and our body language.

One time I flew down to Hobart to present at a seminar. The weather on the day that I flew in, did not look good – heavy dark clouds and by early afternoon the rain was heavy. I met the seminar organiser at the venue, where he was preparing the seating for 60 people who had booked in for the seminar. It was continuing to teem down and I was starting to doubt that anyone would come out in that kind of weather. But the organiser was very optimistic and said quite confidently that most of the people would turn up. And that's exactly what happened! They arrived wearing raincoats, carrying wet umbrellas and smiling as they gradually entered the venue – amazing. Over 50 people came and it was a great night. A reminder for me, how our mindset can influence the outcome.

Here is an everyday situation we commonly deal with – driving into a car park. We can start feeling anxious or annoyed, saying to ourselves – *"I can never find a spot in this car park"* and driving more quickly and missing spots about to become vacant. Or we can say to ourselves as we start driving into the car park – *"The right car spot is waiting for me."* Then driving calmly around and inevitably a spot is waiting for you. I use this all the time. In fact if my grandchildren are in the car with me, they start chanting – *"The right car spot is waiting for us"* and get all excited when one appears.

Also, rather than focussing on what you *'don't want'* or *'can't do'* – turn your thoughts around to what you **'do want'** or what you **'could do'**. Also thinking of the good in your life instead of thinking too much about what you don't have or being envious of others. These little changes help you to think more positively up to 80% of the time, rather than vice versa.

All through our lives we are challenged by people and situations that can affect us in negative ways. We can let these things pull us down – cause us to worry, get angry, lose confidence, get depressed and even age faster. Or we can choose to change our thinking, look at the issues through fresh eyes – find solutions to the problem, look at what is working in our lives, let go of the negative thinking patterns, move on, stay healthy and slow down the ageing process. Positive thinking keeps the mind healthy and can help people to overcome depression.

When you wake up – focus on what you can do, to make the day feel alive and interesting.

When you go to bed – focus on what went well during your day and be thankful.

Catch Your Thoughts - Change Your Thoughts - Change Your Life ☺

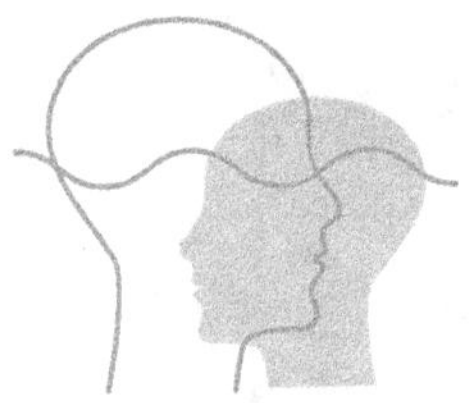

3

Endings and New Beginnings

Major and sometimes dramatic and sudden changes to our lives are emotionally draining and if not dealt with in the right way, can stop people moving on with their lives.

It is not just older workers who retire. Younger sports people are another group who retire from a career dedicated to their particular sport. Michael Phelps, the American Olympic swimmer in his late 20's, who has won a number of gold medals, announced his retirement from his swimming career at the recent London Olympics. He expressed his concern that he had no idea what he was going to do when he stopped swimming. Former Australian athlete, Cathy Freeman retired from her athletic career in 2003 after the Sydney Olympics, aged 30. She said that it took her five years to re-invent herself and find purpose in her life, after giving her whole life to her athletic career.

Entering any new phase of life, requires a letting go of the previous one and there is grief in letting go. I'd like to share with you, a process to handle major changes that I found helpful.

In 1969, psychiatrist Elisabeth Kubler Ross wrote a book called *'Death and Dying'* in which she introduced what has become known as 'The 5 Stages of Grief'. Besides helping people to deal with death, this model has been expanded to help people to handle other major changes/losses in their lives such as — redundancy, ageing, divorce, retirement, relocating, financial loss, natural disasters such as floods and bushfires.

It is important to note that there is no set time frame for each of the five stages. We are all different and some stages may last longer for some people than others. I see it as a roadmap to guide you through a crisis and to eventually see *'the light at the end of the tunnel'* so that you can re-build your life. It takes time to re-group after a major life change. Go with the flow of your emotions, passing through each stage, knowing that you can feel positive again.

I have chosen redundancy as the focus, to show you how to work through the 5 stages of grief, in order to give closure to what *'was'* and prepare for a new beginning.

Surviving Redundancy.

It's interesting to note that 60% - 80% of people from varying age groups have been made redundant at least once in some industries. Redundancy can be a roller-coaster ride. There is expert advice available on your rights and entitlements, which are important to look into. You need to know how long you can survive financially without work. It is important to get financial advice and work out a budget to see you through the period that you are unemployed.

The following section is focused on how to deal with the emotional impact of redundancy. **The 5 Stages of Grief:-**

1. **Denial:** Being told that – *"Your services are no longer required"* can be one of the worst things to be told, especially if it comes out of the blue. You can go numb and the reality of not having a job any longer, can take a few days or even a few weeks to sink in. As a defence mechanism to deal with feelings like shock and embarrassment, it is easy to pretend at first, that it didn't happen and everything is okay. I know of a man who pretended to keep going to work for a few weeks after he was made redundant. Because of his pride, he couldn't bear to tell his family. He would spend the day in the city, walking around, reading the paper, filling in the day till it was time to go home. Eventually, when he felt ready he did tell them.

2. **Anger:** Once the shock wears off, which may take days or weeks, you can start to feel very hurt and rejected, which can lead to feelings of anger. You may be saying things to yourself like – *"It's not fair." "Why has this happened to me? What have I done wrong?"* It is normal to feel anger. Rather than bottling it up, it is important to be able to express it in such a way that it can be resolved. It is very helpful at this point, to be able to talk to someone who can help you deal with the anger – a counsellor, a trusted friend or someone who has survived redundancy. What can be under the feelings of anger are confusion, guilt, diminishing self-confidence and self-worth. By being able to talk to someone, you learn how to manage your feelings, which helps you to move on.

3. **Bargaining:** It is easy to start blaming yourself for being made redundant. *"Perhaps I didn't try hard enough." "I should have worked harder."* Sometimes people have gone back to their workplace and bargained to get their position back – promising

to work harder, longer, etc. The reality is, that there are a number of reasons you could have been made redundant that have nothing to do with your competence. In many cases it may have been because of a company merger, take-over, companies moving jobs offshore, advanced technology, failing profits, poor management. Don't take it personally.

4. **Depression:** You may have started to apply for new positions, with no results. It is easy for despair to take hold and you can start to slide into depression if not dealt with. Spending a lot of time on your own watching TV during the day is a sign that you could be giving up hope. Well-meaning friends may be saying things like *"Time to get over it"* *'Be positive"* *"Build a bridge and move on"* but that is easier said than done if you are feeling depressed. It is important to see a health professional before the depression worsens and your health becomes affected.

Going for a daily walk, or even running or cycling, especially in the mornings, can help to take your mind off your issues and cope better. The exercise can calm you down and clear your head. To make it easier to motivate yourself, think, *"I want to feel better"* rather than thinking *"I don't want to feel depressed."* At first you may need to push yourself to get up and go for a walk, but eventually it will become a habit that will keep you healthy in body, mind and spirit, as was discussed in greater detail in the previous chapter.

Research studies show that regular walking has so many benefits for the physical, mental and emotional body and can improve your mental state to help reduce anxiety. Walking regularly, becomes a good habit that will serve you well through your whole life and help to slow down the ageing process.

5. **Acceptance:** In this final stage, you are coming to terms with your redundancy and getting back on your feet. For

some people this can take up to a year or more, for others it can happen sooner. You are now seeing *'the light at the end of the tunnel'* and have allowed time to grieve the loss. You are finally seeing redundancy as an opportunity to move on in your life. You may now have a different attitude to the importance of a balanced work and personal life.

You are now ready to **'take the plunge'** into new beginnings. You can start this process earlier during the five stages. Review your previous employment. What did you like the most/least about your position? There are a couple of inventories in Chapter 7, that you can complete to help you in this process of re-inventing yourself. Focus on your strengths and think about a different kind of position you could apply for that would utilise those strengths. Get involved in networking to develop contacts. Learn how to prepare a good resume and how to *'sell'* yourself at an interview. Never give up, as you don't know what is around the corner.

Keep yourself active, look after your health, watch your thoughts, get involved in some volunteering which can take your mind off your own problems. Read more about volunteering in Chapter 8. When a new job opportunity does come along you'll feel fitter, healthier and more confident to start afresh.

Col's story – Coming to Terms with Change.

One day six years ago, Col, who was a Bank Manager, was told by his immediate superior, *"I would like to put someone younger in your job."* Col, who was 59 and had worked in the banking industry for 41 years, found this comment very offensive and resigned, rather than being made redundant. He entered retirement earlier than he had planned. In talking to him, I found that he experienced the five stages of grief in his own way.

In the first five years, Col found retirement to be the most difficult time of his life. Suddenly all purpose in life and all the structures and routines were taken away and he was at a loose end as to what to do. His self-esteem was shattered, having always given of his best. After 41 years of working in the banking industry, the regular interaction with co-workers and customers was now replaced with feelings of loneliness and despair. For about 3 years Col felt bitter and wondered what was the purpose of his life. He felt like he had lived to work and now felt like he had retired to die. He became depressed – slept a lot, lost interest in playing golf and stayed indoors a lot.

It took Col five years to come to terms with retired life and it is still evolving. He appreciates the support of his family, likes to go fishing, walks his dog and is now a member of Legacy. He attends the monthly meetings, has been a committee member and enjoys the social interaction. He is now becoming more positive about developing a life after work.

*"Man cannot discover new oceans,
unless he has the courage to lose sight
of the shore." –* Andre Gide

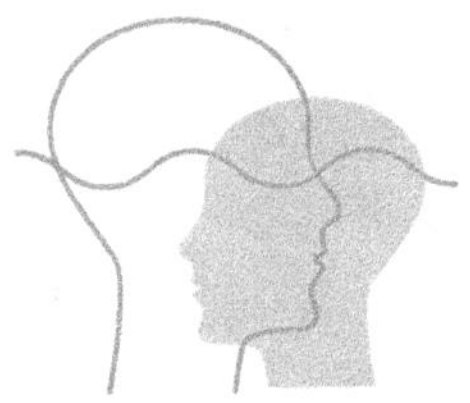

4

Take The Plunge

"Don't wait. The time will never be just right." Napoleon Hill

What are we waiting for? What do we keep putting our lives on hold for? Often, it takes natural disasters and other people's tragedies, to hit home the importance of appreciating life - what is important and what is not that important in the big picture.

Having experienced the deaths of three friends within a period of three months in recent times, has been a big wake-up call. It has made me realise how precious life is and how we don't know when our own time will be up. We have this one life, so let's make the most of it.

At different times in our lives, we can be hesitant to begin a new venture. There may be an element of risk involved, which means stepping out of our comfort zone. We can hold off **taking the plunge** because of our fears and the uncertainty of the outcome. If you have been thinking of doing something different to bring changes into your life, but keep hesitating, ask yourself *'What is the worst thing that could happen?'* Then ask yourself *'What are the benefits if I do take the plunge?'* Has the time come to step outside the box and refresh your life? Listen to your heart, your gut feeling, your intuition – which works best for you.

I remember 24 years ago, standing at a tram stop in Melbourne. I was new to the city and on my way to my first Toastmasters meeting. Those very thoughts I just mentioned, were going through my mind as I waited for the tram. I decided that if I didn't like the meeting, I didn't have to go back, but at least I would have given it a go. As it turned out, I enjoyed the meeting, was made to feel very welcome and joined the Essendon Toastmasters Club. I was an active member for 8 years before we moved away from Melbourne. To think I almost didn't get on the tram! The experiences I had and the skills I learnt, helped me to create my own presentation skills training programs, that have helped many people over the years to overcome their fear of public speaking. It is a wonderful feeling, to watch people benefit and grow from the knowledge and experiences that you are able to share with them.

I'd like to share with you, two stories from people who *'took the plunge'* in different ways and changed their lives for the better as a result.

Elizabeth's story – From Here to There.

A couple of years ago I met a woman called Elizabeth who had just turned 90. She was a happy, lively woman who played ten pin bowling, loved her needlework, did some oil painting, and even though she had learnt to use the computer, sent hand-written letters to her long-time friends in the UK every week.

Elizabeth's husband died after a long illness in 1991 in Western Australia, where they had moved to from the UK 30 years earlier. She was in her mid 70's when he passed away. As well as a son living in Perth, Elizabeth had a daughter living on the north coast of NSW, whom she hadn't seen for a few years. She was going to fly and then decided to step out of her comfort zone and drive herself across the Nullarbor Plain, from one side of the country to the other and just take her time and unwind after the stress of her husband's long illness and passing. Wow – driving all that way on her own in her 70's!

She arrived safely and over the next few weeks, enjoyed her stay with her daughter and grand children and began thinking whether she could move over permanently. On the drive back to WA, Elizabeth had a travelling companion, a dog she had acquired while staying with her daughter. She loved having the dog as her companion, especially when they slept in the car sometimes.

Once back in Perth, she weighed up the pros and cons of staying put or moving over to the east coast. She eventually decided that life was too short to hold back and a few months later, drove all the way back across the Nullarbor, with her dog and a car filled with her belongings. She arrived safely at her daughter's place and has lived happily on the far north coast for the past 18 years. How amazing is that to criss-cross the continent on her own, in her 70's and doing all the driving. And I think, that if I drive from the far north coast down to Sydney in one day, I have done a huge trip on my own!

I caught up with Elizabeth recently, now aged 92. She was recovering from the flu which had knocked her around. She had stopped playing ten pin bowling, a game she had played for more than 30 years. To maintain social contact, she goes to the local club a few times a week, to have coffee and catch up with people. She still does needlework, takes her dog for a daily walk, plays games on the computer and does a bit of gardening.

Elizabeth's philosophy is to keep a positive attitude, smile, not cry when life hands out lemons and helping others makes her feel good. She is glad she 'took the plunge' and made the decision when she did, to move and refresh her life.

Beth's Story –Our New Life.

I retired in 1997 from my position as a rehabilitation aide in the local hospital. My husband had retired before me, so we were both free agents. Each winter we would pack up the caravan and head north towards Queensland. The prospect of cold bones as we got older, was not that appealing. We had such great times caravanning and met lots of wonderful people. Our six children from our two previous marriages, plus 15 grandchildren, all knew that one day we would leave Canberra, but none of us knew when, including ourselves.

On our annual migration north in 2003, we visited friends who lived in an Over 50's Lifestyle Park in Kingscliff, on the far north coast of NSW. They invited us to stay for a BBQ and showed us around the complex. We were very impressed with the great facilities and checked out some houses for sale. We realised that we were at a crossroad in our life. It is one thing to talk about moving north, but quite another thing when it comes to decision time. We both felt we wanted an adventure before it was too late, but would moving north do the trick?

We'd had a few experiences that were motivating us to move. Canberra had been experiencing a drought and then came the bushfires. We had 15 houses burn to the ground around us. What an unbelievable day that was! This made us re-evaluate how we were living our life:- Life can be uncertain – life is precious. Many of our friends had left Canberra when they retired and we felt lonely. My dream ever since childhood was, to one day be a beachcomber. The time had come to move up north and live the dream. Also, two of our children and their families lived up north so we could see more of them.

Time to do the things we were putting off. Moving north to Kingscliff was becoming more desirable every day. We talked about the needs we would have, as we aged, like transport and medical facilities and Kingscliff ticked all the boxes. We were still wondering if we were doing the right thing, so we compiled a list of the advantages and disadvantages of moving. The main disadvantage was leaving our children and grandchildren who still lived in Canberra, but then we realised, that there was no guarantee they would be staying in Canberra.

We decided – YES! We deserved to live our dream, have our adventure and make a new life for ourselves in retirement. Why hold back? Our families were fine with our decision, which was a great relief for us. They were already seeing our new home as a great place to come for a holiday!

It was such a big decision leaving a place where we had lived for 34 years, but 9 years later, it has been the right decision. We have expanded our lives so much and done things we never thought we would do. Some of the activities that my husband and I are involved in at our Park include – singing, concert productions, indoor bowls, patchwork group. We are also involved in activities in the town community – U3A, Lions Club, Probus Club, Dune Care, Life Writing class, Walking group. And we have made lots of new friends. No time to be lonely!

Since moving here 9 years ago, my husband has had two bouts of cancer, but thanks to the great medical care up here, he is now in the best of health. After the first cancer- melanoma, we were motivated to do a trip we had talked about for some time, the Indian-Pacific train trip across the Nullarbor. Three years later, after his prostate cancer, we did another trip we had always wanted to do, travelling to Canada and Alaska. My husband's cancer had given us a wake-up call to live life and not keep putting things off.

We have about 3 trips a year back to Canberra to see our families. It's amazing how much the grandchildren grow between visits. Sometimes the grandchildren fly up in the school holidays to stay with us. Our move has brought us a fuller, richer life, not to mention warmer.

Our attitude is – "Do it while you can, because we don't know what the future holds.

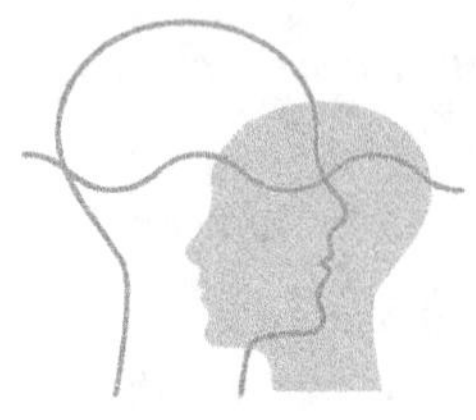

5

Ask and You Will Receive

This would have to be one of the most quoted extracts from the bible. The secret of this simple, yet powerful message, is to focus on what you **do want**, rather than on what you don't want and it can come to you. For example, if you are in a job or a relationship that is causing you to feel unhappy, it is easy to get bogged down in constantly thinking about what is not working, which can keep you stuck in that situation – nothing changes.

If you turn your thinking around and get clearer on what you do want from a job or a relationship, eg. *"I want a boss who is fair and listens to me. I want a partner who is thoughtful and supportive."* Each time you find yourself getting bogged down in the *"I don't want…"* thoughts, you can change to thoughts of what you do want and allow changes for the better to come into your life.

Instead of saying- ***"I don't want to get sick"***, much better to say ***"I <u>want</u> to stay healthy."*** While you stay stuck in thinking about what you don't want, nothing changes.

As you think, so shall it be."

A number of years ago most of my training programs were run in the evenings or at weekends. After a while, I realised that this cut into my social life with family and friends. I kept saying to myself that I didn't want to run courses on week nights and at weekends all the time. But nothing changed. When I started to focus on what I wanted – to run some courses on week days and less on weekends, it was amazing how opportunities for running courses during the week, started to happen. I had started to network with business organisations and this soon opened the door to week day training opportunities.

With money issues, it will work better when you ask for a specific amount, what you need it for and how that can improve your life. Be patient about **how** and **when** it will happen.

I think it's important when you have *'asked and received'* to **express thanks**, as that opens the door for more requests being fulfilled. I have used this process of *'ask and receive'* for a number of years.

I do think that your desires need to be realistic. If you say you want to win the lottery and you don't win, it would be easy to say *"This doesn't work."* It is more effective to focus on what you actually want the money for. Is the money for a new car, new home, travel?

Focus on personal issues in your everyday life, asking for guidance with what you really want. Then it can manifest, sometimes quickly, other times not so quickly. It's amazing how things start to unfold to bring your desire into reality, if you believe and trust that it **can** happen and that **you deserve a great life**.

Be careful what you ask for. I know a woman who years ago, kept saying she wanted to marry a rich man and eventually she did. He was wealthy but he was also a rather mean and nasty person. The marriage didn't last long and she was wiser because of it. In hindsight (which is a wonderful thing!) she could have said that she wanted to marry a man who was wealthy and also kind and loving. What a better marriage that would have been!

The 6 steps to empower your chances of receiving what you ask for:-

1. **<u>Think it</u>** – Get clear in your mind, the details of what you are asking for. Your thoughts create a mental blue print of what you are asking for. *"I would love to go overseas. I really want to lose weight. I want to improve my tennis game.*

2. **<u>See it</u>** – Picture in your mind, what it is you want and keep enhancing it. Create a board where you can hang pictures of what you want or do your own drawings.

3. **<u>Feel it</u>** – Important to feel a connection with your heart, that this desire is strong and feels right for you and is for your highest good. Feel that you deserve it.

4. **<u>Write it down</u>** – It has been proven that when we actually write down what we want with all the details, it increases the chances of your desire coming into reality. We have moved a few times in the last 25 years and I found this process of writing down in detail, the kind of features we wanted in our new place, very helpful. It was amazing how many of the features we did get each time!

5. **<u>Say it</u>** – Verbalise your desire, by reading aloud each day, what you have written. This also strengthens your intention.

6. **<u>Believe it</u>** – You must ask, believing that you deserve it. Sometimes deep-seated beliefs can keep us stuck in old patterns that we 'don't deserve', which can block or slow down what we are asking for, coming into our life.

I think it's better **not** to tell others what you are asking for, because the last thing you want is a negative person to tell you "It won't work. It's a silly idea. You're dreaming!" and sabotage what you are trying to do. Don't take other people's negative comments on board.

Now relax and trust. Just follow the 6 steps every day and *'let go'* of **how** or **when** it is going to happen. I also add, *"This or something better now comes into my life."*

Be mindful that you don't slide into old, negative thought patterns. If you are asking for abundance to flow into your life, then don't think about never having enough money. You can't expect prosperity to come into your life, if you keep thinking about not having enough money.

"Where your focus goes, your energy flows."

When I was writing my first book, I used the *'6 step'* process. I believed that I could run seminars in conjunction with my book; I visualised working with financial organisations; I began creating my seminar topic; I pictured myself presenting in front of groups around the country – all before I had actually finished writing my book! I felt a very strong desire to do this. I have found, that when your desire for what you are asking, feels like a burning desire in your heart, the 6 steps are easy to do. And that is what eventually happened, even though at the time I had no idea how it would happen. I have presented at over 200 seminars around Australia with various financial groups. I received what I asked for!

Imagine going down to the edge of the ocean beach. You take a bucket and fill a large tub with a six bucketfuls of water. It makes no difference to the level of the ocean. Or you pour six cupfuls of water into the tub. The level of the ocean hasn't changed. The six cups of water would hardly fill the tub compared to the six bucketfuls. The Universe is abundant, so why settle for less, when you can have more! What have you got to lose?

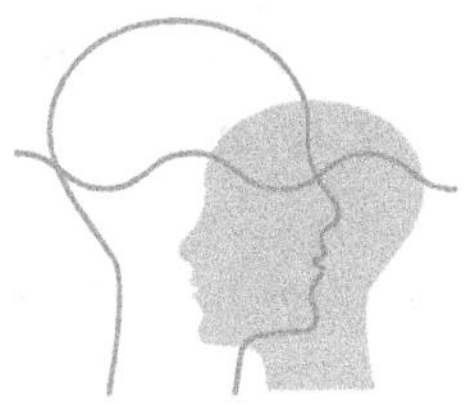

6

Breath of Calm

I would like to share with you, a simple yet powerful technique, that doesn't cost any money, and can be carried out anytime and anywhere. This powerful, yet easy technique involves breathing – something we do automatically every moment of our lives without thinking about it. What is unique about our breath is that, even though it is an involuntary function of the body, we do have control over it. How easy is that!

For thousands of years, yoga and meditation have taught, that by controlling your breath, you can improve your health, think more clearly, and reduce stress. When we get stressed, feel angry, worried or anxious, our rate of breathing increases.

To slow down and deepen your breathing, there are different techniques available, which you can use yourself anytime. The one that is easy to use and works for me is belly breathing. This technique can help to still our busy minds and restore clearer, calmer thinking.

Belly breathing switches on the parasympathetic nervous system, the calming part of our nervous system:-

1. Breathe in slowly through your nostrils, mouth closed, to the steady count of 3. Feel the belly expanding, but <u>not</u> your shoulders rising. You can check this by resting your hand, palm down, gently on your lower belly as you breathe in.
2. Hold the breath for the count of 3.
3. Then breathe out slowly through your mouth, to the count of 3. Keep your hand on your belly so that you can feel it going down as you exhale. Repeat this cycle at least 6 times. It is easy for the mind to wander, when you first start doing this, As you keep practising, you will find it easier to stay focused on the breathing.

The mind can only focus on one thing at a time, so when you focus on the counting, your mind can't be thinking of something else at the same time. You will find that after a few breaths, you will develop a steady rhythm. Whether you are at work or at home, you can use this breathing technique to calm yourself down, when you find yourself feeling uptight about something.

The belly breathing technique is very helpful and easy to use when you have difficulty going to sleep. Rather than resorting to sleeping tablets, this is a less invasive way to get a good night's sleep. When you go to bed thinking about issues and feel restless, place your hands on your belly and do the breathing technique as described earlier. To calm the busy or worried mind ready for sleep, use the counting process or a special word. You could say *'in'* on the in-breath and *'out'* on the out-breath. If your mind goes back to thinking about your problem, just re-focus on the counting of the in and out breath. Or count sheep! By focusing on the counting or words, the mind starts to calm down and before long you can fall asleep. A benefit of good sleep is that it can help to slow down the ageing process.

An interesting article I read some time ago and has stuck in my mind, is that the word **'calm'** has an immediate and quite noticeable calming effect on people. Author, Paul Wilson, conducted a study many years ago on the physiological impact of words used as mantras for meditation. Except for those using personal mantras, the simple word *'calm'* came out on top. Users found this the most calming and pleasing word for use in meditation. Great athletes before the beginning of an event, create a state of *'inner calm'* in their minds using the breath.

I love my daily walk which I combine at times, with the breathing technique. Just being outdoors in the fresh air away from the computer, adds to the power of this process. As I'm walking along at a steady pace, I do my belly breathing. What I find makes it even more powerful, is to say a word in your mind, with each in-breath, something you want to strengthen in yourself, and when you breath out, say a word silently to yourself, something you want to eliminate. The words you use can relate to an issue you are experiencing at the time. For example, as I breathe in, I say to myself – *'Breathe in FAITH'* and when I breathe out, I say to myself –*'Breathe out FEAR'*. I find this very powerful. You could say, *'Breathe in CALM'* - *'Breathe out ANGER'*. Sometimes it may take quite a few in /out breaths to diffuse any anger you may be feeling, but eventually if you persist calmly with the belly breathing, you can feel the tension dissolving. Much healthier than holding that anger in! Just think of what quality you want to strengthen and what you want to reduce.

Hawaiians use the word *'Aloha'* to breathe fully. Breathe in on *'Alo'* and out on *'ha'*. While doing it, you are breathing in love as *'Aloha'* means *'love'* as well as the commonly known *'hello'*. Try it.

Before you head off on a walk or start the breathing process, make a pact with yourself, to let go of thinking about stressful issues that may be occurring in your life and allow the power of the breathing process I have just described, to heal and energise you.

When I get home from my walks, I feel clearer in my mind, more relaxed and more energetic. Sometimes as I am doing this breathing process on my walks, an answer will flash into my mind about something I have been trying to sort out. I do believe that as you let go of your busy thoughts and allow the breathing technique to deepen your breathing and calm your mind, the answers you need come to you!

I urge you to start doing this breathing technique on a daily basis, walking, sitting or lying down. Create a habit and you can start noticing some of the benefits I mentioned earlier. It takes about two weeks to create a new habit, so be patient with yourself as you gradually get into the habit of using this breathing process to think more clearly, reduce stress and improve your health.

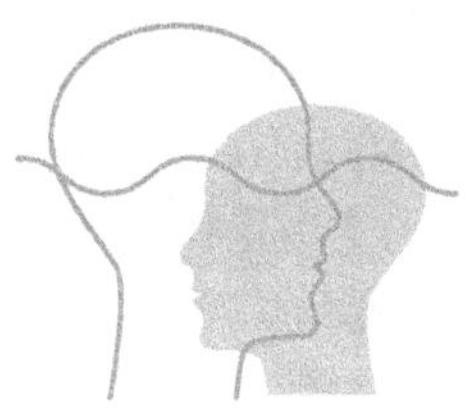

7

The Changing Face of Retirement

Just over 100 years ago, the *'Old Age Pensions Act'* was introduced in the UK and in Australia for those over 65 years. One hundred years ago the average life expectancy was around 55 years. Not many people lived long enough to even get the pension. Back then about 34,000 people received the pension which was ten shillings a week. In 1950, there were 664,000 Australians aged 65 and over.

Today the Age Pension is paid to over 2 million people. The extension of life expectancy imposes a greater financial burden on the Australian Government of supporting more people of pension age. As a way of starting to deal with this crisis, the government plans to raise the pension age to 67 by 2024. They are even talking of raising the pension age to 70. It's interesting to note that if the age pension had kept pace with our changing life expectancy, it would now start at around 80!

Today the average life expectancy is around 80 years, with an increase in the number of people living over 100. There are over 3,000 Australians over the age of 100 and this number is expected to increase to 78,000 by 2055. Australians have the second-longest life expectancy in the world, after Japan.

Of the 22.7 million people living in Australia today, four million are the 'baby boomers' born between 1946 – 1961. By 2030 it is predicted that there will be more people over 65 than under 14. In the 1950's, 35% of the population were children. Today, about 20% of the population are children. If this figure continues to decrease, there will be a problem with finding enough skilled workers in the future.

No wonder baby boomers don't like the **'R'** word! As they are living 20-30 years longer, to still have 65 symbolising *'old age'* is so out-dated. Today's baby boomers are healthier, more educated, and have a good third of their lives still ahead of them. We have so many **more choices** than previous generations, on what to do with this next stage of our lives. Having all these choices – whether to make a tree/sea change, buy a motor home, travel, keep working - the list goes on, making it difficult to decide what you really want to do. Will it suit your lifestyle? Will it fit in with your long-term budget, especially as we are living longer?

This is why it is becoming just as important to start thinking about life planning in conjunction with financial planning, so that you know how to spend your time without spending all your money.

The global financial crisis in 2008 and recent economic downturns have affected the decision to retire earlier. Many people lost money in their super funds, so they are a lot more cautious about retiring too soon. A growing number of baby boomers are continuing to work after 65, some continuing in their full-time positions, others working part-time. A recent National Seniors survey found that, since the Global Financial Crisis four years ago, 50% of the over-50's baby boomers have decided to delay retirement and 75% have cut back on their spending. The retirement dream for baby boomers is moving further down the track.

The face of retirement is changing in a number of ways and the baby boomers are at the forefront of the changes. I will discuss in further detail, in the following chapters, how to deal with these changes in the different areas of our lives.

Changing Times in the Workplace.

The workplace is also changing because of an ageing population. The main factors underlying population ageing, are the increased life expectancy and reducing fertility rates. This came from a study conducted by the Queensland Government. It is going to become harder for organisations to maintain an adequate workforce in the coming years as more baby boomers start to retire and less of the younger generation are entering the workforce.

By 2020, it has been estimated that 85% of the growth in the labour market will come from the over 45year olds.

Unfortunately age discrimination is still played out. Some businesses have a mentality that older workers are 'getting past their use-by-date'. Instead of getting rid of valuable workers in their 50's and 60's and losing their skills, organisations need to think about the benefits of keeping mature workers in the workforce.

The good news is, that new figures just released, show that mature workers over 55 in Australia, account for 17.4% of the workforce, as of August 2012, an increase of about 76,200 since a year ago.

When we were in Auckland, New Zealand earlier this year, we visited the Sky Tower. From the top, you get the most stunning views of the region surrounding Auckland. We heard the story of Warren Green, a 62 year old respected crane expert, who came out of retirement, to show others how to get the crane down, once the Sky Tower was finished. No one else could work out how to do it. It's good that the knowledge and expertise of an older worker is respected.

Who likes to have their competence in the workplace judged purely by their birth date? It can be quite humiliating to be made redundant solely for this reason, if in fact, you are very capable in your role at work and enjoy your position. Thankfully there are organisations that do value older workers and have created **flexible work arrangements** to keep their skills and knowledge.

Bunnings is a great example of a business that values older employees for their skills and knowledge and offer flexible work arrangements. If working parents of pre-schoolers can get flexible work arrangements, so should mature-age workers.

The ideal way to ease into retirement, stay healthy and enjoy life in retirement, is to have the option to keep working with a more flexible structure. A study in America found that 76% of mature workers said that flexible work arrangements were essential if they were to be retained longer. It is a win–win situation for both the employer and employee.

Some ideas for creating flexibility at work and helping mature age employees to 'shift down' while still maintaining their skills and experience, could be:- part-time hours, job sharing, fifth day off using accrued long service leave, retraining for a different position in the workplace, mentoring younger employees. A win-win for both employers and employees.

There are many benefits of **retaining - retraining - recruiting** mature-age employees, by incorporating more flexible work arrangements:-

- Lower absenteeism and turnover rates.
- Strong work ethic and employer loyalty.
- Experience, wisdom and dependability.
- A healthy and diverse organisational culture spanning all age groups.

- The company is not losing the expertise that would be costly to replace.
- The employees still feel valued.
- Productivity is successfully maintained.

Many older employees, who aren't ready to fully retire, are moving into a new role, that may pay less, but can be more personally rewarding and less pressure than their previous full-time position. Studies have shown that half the men who went back to work after retirement, did so because they wanted to, usually because they were bored with life in retirement.

When is the right time to stop working? What interests do you have, that you can develop once you do retire? How much money is enough for you to retire on? Do you _want_ to keep on working or do you feel you _have_ to? How is your health? Best to retire while still healthy, rather than 'burnt-out' from staying too long in the workforce.

Studies have shown that less than 30% of people retire when they plan to. Redundancy, ill health, a work place closing down, are some of the things that can push people into sudden retirement they weren't ready for. That's why it is important to have some ideas already, on how you will live life once you stop working.

Handling unexpected retirement: Maintaining an attitude of hope in the face of sudden, unplanned retirement, can be quite difficult at first and it can be easy to become depressed. It is important to seek support for – career planning advice, outplacement services, counselling, financial advice on entitlements – choose the best option for your needs. As one door closes, see a new door opening. See this as a new beginning, a new opportunity to re-invent yourself – rather than staying stuck in the past or full of regrets. That is why it is important to seek support.

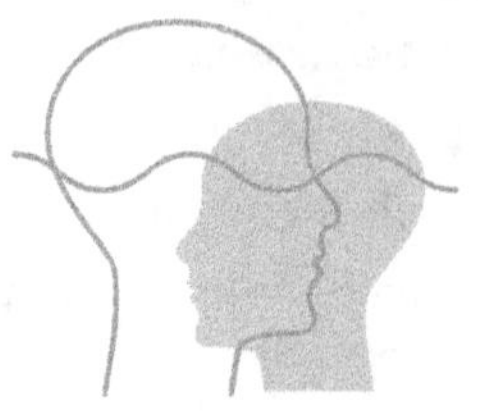

8

Re-invent Yourself

During your work life, you were identified by your role – Bob the Builder, Tina the Teacher, David the Doctor, Mick the Mechanic, Anna the Athlete and the list goes on. This title during your work life, created a sense of identity and a feeling of self-worth. For men in particular, this loss of identity, can be distressing, not having the familiar routines anymore to fill their days.

It is important not to define yourself by your work role and to realise that when you retire or are made redundant, you are still the person inside, that you were before the work role. But now you have a wealth of life skills, work skills and wisdom, which you can turn into many other directions and use to enrich your own life, as well as the lives of others in the community. Retirement can actually be an important part of your life. The inventory at the end of this chapter can help you to get back in touch with what you are good at.

To deal with this loss of identity, following is a self-inventory that you can use to re-discover your true self, after full-time work. The more clearly you understand your real needs, the easier it is to let go of excess baggage from your past.

Who Am I?

- What makes me feel good about myself?
- What would I like to do better?
- What interests do I enjoy?
- Who do I feel comfortable being around?
- What is important to me?
- What stops me doing what I really want to do?
- What would it take to make my life more interesting?

It is interesting the number of people, mainly men, who have come up after a seminar and told me, that because they have been so busy working all those years, they are scared of retirement, as they don't know what they'll do. It is an issue that needs thought, ideally before retirement starts.

A. One man I spoke with at a seminar, already has a new role in mind for life after full-time work. He is an accountant and in his spare time he upholsters furniture. This is a hobby that he is going to develop into a small business when he retires. As he shared his vision with me, he spoke with excitement about the new opportunities ahead of him.

B. A woman I know of, retired from teaching and a couple of years later, turned her passion for gardening into a successful landscape business. Another woman, a retired pharmacist, was given a knitting machine by an elderly neighbour. The retired pharmacist developed quite a passion for learning how to use the machine and creating knitted articles. She now travels around the country, showing other women how to use knitting machines. She also enters her knitted items in the Royal Easter Show and wins prizes.

C. On a trip to a northern Queensland city to present at a seminar, I travelled from the airport in a taxi driven by a 64 year old man. After he retired, he missed the social interaction of his former workplace, now that he lived on property out of town. Driving a taxi three afternoons a week, gave him the opportunity to chat to people and earn some extra money for his hobby – stuffing crocodiles!

What these three stories highlight is, that when you think outside the square and get in touch with doing something you really enjoy, you can live a happier, healthier, more meaningful life.

Start re-inventing yourself. Didn't you always want to be your own boss? Do something you would really like to do. Use skills you already have, learn new ones, do volunteer work, the list is endless. Your local newspaper or the internet can give you ideas for activities you can do.

Following is an inventory to tick **what you are good at**. Expand on the items in the inventory that use your skills and talents. No one is good at everything, but some things you might do very well. Start ticking: √

- Great sense of humour
- Organizing things
- Helpful
- Listening
- Environmentally aware
- Useful in emergencies
- Playing a musical instrument

- Playing sport
- Enjoying a hobby
- Fixing things
- Enjoy conversation
- Getting along well with others
- Cooking
- Gardening
- Driving
- Learning new things
- Managing a budget
- Drawing and painting
- Writing
- Managing the house
- Active committee member

By completing this inventory, you may be pleasantly surprised at the skills you could use to help others. You could also tap into some things you'd like to learn, now that you have more time on your hands.

Greg's story – Sudden Retirement

"I am one of those 65% of Australians to whom retirement came unexpectedly. I was a high school music teacher and also worked as a professional musician and piano tutor in my spare time. I worked seven days a week for many years. Last year I suffered 'teacher burnout' and was diagnosed with depression.

I had planned to work for another 5 years till I reached 67, before I planned to retire, but that was not to be. For years I used to dread the idea of retirement and wondered how I would ever cope.

Fortunately, I had taken the time earlier that year, before my 'burn out' to do two positive things in relation to thinking of my future retirement, which at the time I believed was still a long way off.

- *Devised a list of the Top 50 things I could do in retirement.*
- *Began one of the volunteer activities that I had listed – Playing the piano at the local hospital as part of the 'Arts in Health' program, even though I hadn't retired yet.*

These two actions have already been a great help to me, on my road to recovery. Gradually, I will put into action, other activities from my Top 50 list, to create my new life in retirement."

Greg's inventory contains 50 activities that use skills and talents he has developed during his life, and now gives him a whole range of interesting ventures to look forward to.

Some of the things on Greg's Top 50 list are:- learn to cook, research his family history, volunteer at the local school, write a text book to help music teachers, learn to play other musical instruments, compose music, become a musical director of a theatre company, travel overseas, to name a few.

Why not start writing your own **Top 50 list** of activities that use your skills and talents that you have developed during your lifetime. Gradually keep adding to the list as you think of new ideas. Then over time, tick off the activities as you do them. You may be amazed what you come up with and what you can end up achieving.

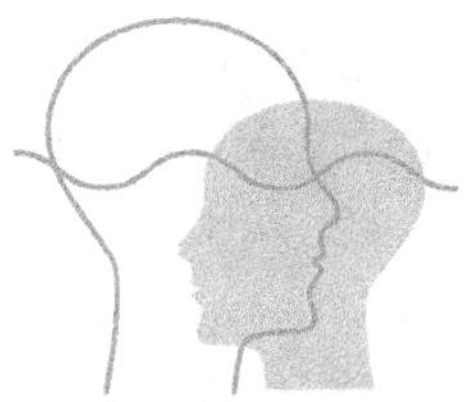

9

Service to Others

"I don't know what your destiny will be, but one thing I know – the only ones among you who will be truly happy, are those who will have sought and found how to serve." - Albert Schweitzer

The beginning of 2011 was a challenging time in many parts of Australia – massive floods and bushfires. A reminder of the power of nature and how little power we humans have, to stop nature's disasters, despite all our modern technology. These disasters and similar ones in other years, have tested the human spirit.

Something wonderful that came out of the Queensland flood crisis, was the amazing community spirit, of the many people who came forth to help thousands of flood victims in a myriad of ways. What came through time and time again, from those affected by the floods, was the comment, that the people in their lives mattered much more than their belongings.

Research has shown that to keep in good health, besides keeping physically fit and eating well, we need to maintain regular, direct social contact with others. When someone goes through a major life change like redundancy, a relationship ending or retirement, it can be easy to withdraw from the company of others and slide into depression. To make the effort to get out there and help others less fortunate, can take your mind off your own problems and help you adjust to a new stage of your life while helping others.

Being of service to others can be very rewarding on a number of levels:- feeling useful, helping others less fortunate, belonging to your community, making a difference, meeting new people and developing new friendships.

Thirty-five years ago, before we had computers and the internet, my husband joined a service club called Apex and for 13 years it was a wonderful way for us to meet people and become part of a new community more easily. I joined Toastmasters and Rotary over the years. These days my husband is a member of Lions – still a great way to meet new people, get involved in service projects, network and enjoy social activities.

Service to others has a number of benefits as I mentioned earlier. Check out service clubs and volunteer groups in your local community that you could become involved in. Go to a couple of meetings and see if it is for you. Try other groups till you find the one that suits you. It is easy to say – *"I'm too busy."* Decide on a realistic commitment of time that you can contribute to projects. Review the benefits I listed earlier – it's a win-win situation for all. The various groups my husband and I have been associated with over the years, have included people still working, young people and retired people – a great cross-section of the community. When you move to a new area to live, joining service clubs and volunteering organisations, is a great way to quickly get involved in the local community, meet people and make new friends.

I would like to share **Sue's story** about volunteering:-
"As a volunteer for Meals on Wheels for the past 20 years, I have been privileged to be part of their organization. During the first 14 years, I was a meal deliverer at two separate services in two different towns. Being a volunteer, helped me to make a connection to our new community, when my husband and I moved there. While we were running a small business, I was able to be of service, at times when they needed me.

Down the track, at about the time we were selling our business and my husband was ready to retire, the manager of our local Meals on Wheels service, offered me the opportunity to co-ordinate a new program, to be run in conjunction with the meal deliveries. This program is a social support program, helping to bring elderly people together, who live on their own. This program has been very successful and I have made many new friends among the other volunteers.

Working on a part-time basis with Meals on Wheels, allows me to pursue my other interests, mainly playing golf, walking on the beach and staying in touch with my family and friends. This mix of activities, help to keep me fit, emotionally and physically."

When you retire, a wonderful way to give service, is to share the skills and knowledge you developed in your working life and **mentor** younger people and prepare them for their career paths. I've spoken with men at retirement seminars who come up and tell me that once they retired, they felt they had lost their value as a person, which is so sad to hear. What I suggest to them is to sit down and write down all the things they feel they can do well and to keep adding to the list. It's surprising what some of them come up with after they have done this list. Review the *'What am I good at'* inventory in the previous chapter.

Abraham Maslow says that one of the key needs of human beings is **purpose.** A sense of purpose delivers a feeling of achievement and fulfilment. This is crucial to achieving one's own unique potential. When you align your skills and talents with your passion and use these together, to serve some kind of need in the community, then you are well on the way to living a great life.

The next step is to seek out organisations and schools, where you can offer your time and expertise to help others. Another outlet to share your skills, is to become a volunteer tutor at a U3A centre near you. The University of the Third Age is a worldwide movement that began in France in 1973, to offer a variety of programs for people over the age of 50 years, who want to keep learning new things and keep their brains active. The tutors are all volunteers. As well as learning something new or being a volunteer tutor, you are also mixing socially and meeting new people.

It's lovely to give and receive gifts on our birthday and at Christmas, but there are many benefits of giving of our time and life experiences to benefit others. **Volunteering** is a *'win-win'* for all concerned – the receiver and the giver. What may not always be noticed are the benefits of giving, especially how beneficial it is for your own health and well–being. Many studies show that the *'helper's high'* creates a sense of warmth and satisfaction, that comes from helping to improve the life of another.

Professor Stephen Post says that – *"The' high' occurs partly because focusing on others, causes a shift from our unhealthy preoccupation with ourselves and reduces the stress-related wear and tear on the body and soul."*

Some more facts about how giving will benefit you: -

- It has been found that people who volunteer have lower levels of depression.
- People who volunteer are more satisfied with their lives, have a stronger will to live, have less anxiety and fewer physical symptoms caused by psychological conditions.
- Older people who volunteer tend to live longer. Giving is good for the heart because it stimulates the production of the hormone oxytocins which protects us from hardening

of the arteries, dilates our blood vessels, reduces blood pressure, and may help the heart regenerate after damage.

- The human body is said to be at its best and healthiest when we are kind and giving.

Go to www.dosomethingnearyou.com.au to find out what volunteering opportunities are available in your area.

The common thread in many studies is that the greatest benefits come from giving on a regular basis. Simple gestures like a weekly visit to an elderly person who lives on their own or is in a nursing home will do it – as long as you do it regularly. A few years ago we lived in a country town where, for 15 months I used to visit a lovely 84 year old Irish woman, who was bedridden after having lived an active life for many years. I visited her most Fridays for an hour or so in the nursing home where she was now living. Even though she was physically impaired, her mind was strong and we used to have some interesting conversations during those 15 months before she passed away. I treasure those memories of my visits with her.

Some more volunteering activities could be:- helping an elderly neighbour each week with their shopping or driving them to an appointment; being a retail volunteer one day a week at a local charity shop; helping people with a disability. You can Google volunteer organisations and look up your local newspaper to find out more information.

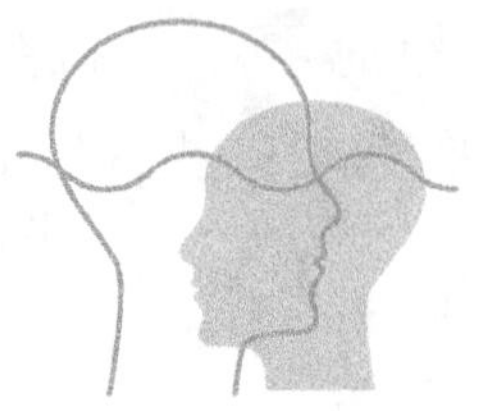

10

"Till Death Us Do Part."

'Till death us do part' – These words are in the wedding vow, for making a commitment for life between a newly wedded couple. It originated in the Book of Common Prayer back in 1662, to be used in marriage services in England. Back then most people didn't live beyond 40, so the typical lifespan of a marriage then was about 20 years.

How times have changed! Today with more people reaching 100, a marriage could last 80 years! In fact, my husband's parents who are both in their early 90's, celebrated their 70th wedding anniversary this year. My husband's parents are of the generation where the husband's role was seen as that of the good provider and the wife's role was seen as the good homemaker and good mother. If you performed those roles well, you were expected to be satisfied with those roles. Personal happiness was less important. Very few women from that generation had a career and divorce was uncommon.

My husband and I married in the late 1960's. Things had already started to change. We baby boomers were at the turning point of major changes in married life. I had a teaching career and more women were developing careers in other areas. When we had our first baby, there was no paid maternity leave, but I could resume my teaching position after 6 months. I was more fortunate than some other women, who were in positions where they had to resign when they became pregnant. In that period, our husbands had grown up in households where their mother stayed home and did all the cooking and cleaning and their father was the sole income provider. Because more women were now working, we had different expectations, such as expecting the husband to share the house duties. Because we were out in the workforce, contributing to the community, mixing with people, making decisions and earning an income, we were no longer prepared to carry out the role of the good mother and the good housekeeper on our own, without support.

By the end of the 1970's, women's liberation was fighting for the rights of women. Paid maternity leave came in and divorce became a solution if a marriage was no longer working. It's interesting to note that the divorce rate in the 50-60's age group has doubled in the past 20 years. A recent American study calls it *'The Gray Divorce Revolution'*. Because we are living longer, the norm of marriage as a lifelong institution is weakening.

As people move into the 50-60's age group, it is a chance to reflect on the prospect of spending another 20-30 years with the same person. The marriage may be okay, but not particularly satisfying. People today question things more than earlier generations. Some marriages hang on for the sake of the children. When they eventually leave home, things can become unstuck. Relationships can break down when issues creep into a relationship as a result of people growing apart. People change over time, perhaps not as compatible as they may have been; not co-operating or compromising; not spending time together; meeting other people; not having anything in common anymore. Re-igniting the flame can be heavy going, especially when over the years, you have settled into routines that can be very predictable.

Meryl Streep, the 63-year-old actress who has starred in some great movies over the years, boasts one of the most enduring marriages in Hollywood. She has been married to her husband for 34 years and they have four grown children. Her tips for a lasting and happy marriage are, *"Stay alert and alive to each other, speak and be heard, break patterns and don't become complacent."*

Retirement can have a big impact on relationships. For many years you may have been used to the routine of one or both partners at work during the week and mainly seeing each other in the evenings and on the weekends. Or you may have been in a partnership where one partner worked away from home for days at a time or did shiftwork. Many couples don't realise how daunting it can be, to be suddenly together 24/7. It's easy to get under each other's feet. In fact, I've had people come up to me at seminars and say they don't want to retire yet, because they are scared of spending too much time with their partner. It has been easy with a busy work life and raising a family, to put issues on the back-burner.

Now, being in each other's space more often, can either give you the opportunity, to either rekindle your relationship, or widen the 'cracks'. Some couples can't wait to have more time together. Others not. Some of the issues that can arise from spending too much time together are:- sharing tasks around the home, respecting each other's time for privacy, time for your own interests.

Another situation to be mindful of when spending a lot of time together, is when travelling on long trips in a caravan. Brenda, a former neighbour, was a friendly, chatty person, while her husband was a man of very few words. When he retired, they set off on what was to be a six month trip up to the top end of Australia. As those of you who have travelled around the country know, you can travel for hundreds of kilometres at times, with little change in the scenery. Brenda found it increasingly stressful, sitting for hours next to a man who didn't engage in conversation. In the end, they returned home three months earlier than planned. When one partner is the silent type, it may be better to consider a trip with a group, where you have others to chat with.

The findings of the *'Relationships Indicators Survey'* carried out in Australia in 2008, listed communication difficulties (37%) and stress about money issues (35%) as the main causes of a relationship breakdown. The survey found that the reasons why older couples, those over 50 separate are:-

- People only stayed together because of the children – 34%
- They had grown apart – 32%
- Wanted a change – 26%
- Midlife crisis – seeing life as too short, to stay stuck in a marriage that was no longer satisfying.

My husband and I separated in our early 40's after seventeen years of marriage and three children. We were apart for nearly four years and we can both look back and see it as a big learning curve in our lives. It was also a period in which I did a lot of personal development and went on to create my own training programs which I loved doing. We never got to the stage of getting divorced, but did get back together again four years later. We started life in a new town, and have since made a return sea change to our former home town and my husband has now retired.

For the past 25 years that we have been back together, we have much better communication and resolve issues before they escalate. If you keep hitting a brick wall in your communication, you can do what we did, years ago when we re-united and that is to get some counselling. Having a trained listener was so helpful. The counsellor helped us to listen properly to each other so that we could resolve issues.

Suppressing anger and bottling things up, can damage your health. It's not, whether or not you argue, but how you do it that counts. If you learn to express your anger and resolve conflict with your partner, your stress levels drop and you can live a longer, happier life.

I find that going on a walk can be a good way to talk things over. There is something about being out in the fresh air and walking as you talk, that keeps the discussion more friendly. Mind you, we still have our moments! As I've mentioned before, the 80/20 rule is a good guide for your relationship. If you are getting on 80% of the time that's great – better than only getting on 20% of the time. No one's perfect.

All relationships have issues of some kind. Most can be solved with open communication. A good heart-to-heart talk can clear the air, as long as you are both on the same wave length. Someone once said that men only hear 1 in 6 words spoken to them. Male and female thought processes can work differently. Men tend to internalise their thoughts, while women are more verbal and this means that we tend to go on longer, till the man says, *"Get to the point, stop going on and on."* Because men keep their thoughts more to themselves, they can forget to include other people in their decisions.

Like the man who travelled a lot with his work and all he wanted to do when he retired, was potter around the garden and go fishing. His wife on the other hand, had stayed at home and had visions of finally being able to travel together when her husband retired. This didn't come out, till the couple were in the office of their financial planner (who told me this story). He suddenly found himself caught in the middle of an explosive eruption, as the couple started yelling at each other about their conflicting desires.

Another communication problem that can happen is when, what one person is saying, is misconstrued by the other. Here's a **story** I hope you enjoy – The husband is at the bar, drowning his sorrows when his mate comes in. *"What's wrong?"* he asks. *"Mate, I can't figure out women,"* he said. *"Why?"* *"Well I came home and there's a note on the fridge from the missus saying: It's not working. I'm off to my mother's,"* the husband said. *"I open the fridge, the light comes on, the beers are cold, it all seems fine. Can't work out why she thought it wasn't working!"*

All the more reason to practise effective communication and listening skills in particular! Listening is so important as misunderstandings can lead to tension, arguments, distance, stress, hurt feelings. If not resolved, can eventually lead to divorce. As money issues are one of the main reasons for partnership breakdowns, good communication can help with formulating a financial plan, based on openness and compromise on goals and expectations, that will lead to much better outcomes and less stress in the relationship.

Communication and relationship difficulties can be **barriers to a good sexual relationship.** It's hard to be close when you have negative feelings toward the other person. Making the time to talk openly and share your feelings can lead to better intimacy and sex. An advantage of mature age sex, as reported in a UK study, suggested that an active sex life can increase longevity. Worth also checking out the remedies available to spice up your sex life! My husband still has a smile on his face, after we ate a bowl of fresh mussels one night, during our New Zealand trip!

A further study done in the UK, gives the following **7 Secrets to a Happy Relationship** (besides a good sex life!)

- **Full body hugs** are proven to stimulate endorphins that help you bond with the person you are hugging. It is also important to be able to show physical affection, without it being sexual. If there has been an issue, it is good to be able to go up and give your partner a body hug and make peace.

- **Keep lines of communication open** – It is easy to drift apart if there are long periods of silence. Regular talks keep you connected, which is what a relationship is about. Accepting that we are all different and respecting each other's differences.
- **Learn to simply enjoy each other's company**, without always needing to be with other people.
- **Go on a special date** once a month helps bonding. It doesn't always mean going out to dinner. It can be going on a bike ride and taking a picnic hamper.
- **Romantic gestures** can be a win-win for both people. The pleasure the person receives by doing the gesture and the pleasure the recipient receives. It can be flowers, but also carrying out a task without being asked to do it.
- **Share housework** without being asked.
- **Have separate nights out occasionally** to maintain your own identity, not taking each other for granted and show that you are happy to come home.

> *"An archaeologist is the best husband any woman can have: the older she gets, the more interested he is in her." –* Agatha Christie

I do think it is worth doing what it takes, to put the spark back into a relationship that has become bland. With any relationship that is becoming negative and you find yourself mainly focusing on what is not working, here is a tip that helps me get back on track. With paper and pen, find a quiet space and write down all the good qualities you can think of in that person. It may take a while because you may be too caught up in what's not working. Write down any little thing that is a positive. Then write a list of the issues that are causing the tension in your relationship with that person.

Are there any things in that list, that in the big picture are not that important, like doing things differently to you around the house? Even after being married for over 40 years, my husband can shift me out of my grumpy moments by making me laugh, which is important in a relationship. It can help me to put back into perspective, an issue that I may have been making a big deal about, that in the big picture was not that important.

Put the list away and go for a walk to clear your head. When you feel ready, go back to the two lists. What are the qualities that you do value? If things still aren't working after your efforts, then you may want to get some counselling. If all else fails, then it may be time to let go and move on. Suggestions for improving your communication skills are given in the next chapter.

There are couples who do stay together **till death does part them**. Couples who have been through the highs and lows together, shared many years of intimacy, had children, had dramas, resolved difficult issues and then one of them passes away due to illness or injury or old age. As we age, death is something we have to face though we don't want to. It can be tough and the support of family and friends is good to have, as you move on with your life in new directions.

Whether you are widowed, divorced or a single person, there are avenues out there, to start a new stage of your life. It is so important to maintain social contact. I met a woman at a computer course I was attending. She was 79 and her partner was 92. They were both widowed when they met at Bingo five years ago and moved in together. She is enjoying her life, having the companionship of her new partner and still doing her own thing as well. Another couple met in a retirement village and got married. Another older woman, has 'sleep-overs' with her boyfriend, but prefers to live in her own place.

You can visit websites like 'Relationships Australia' that offer opportunities to meet prospective partners. The age group that is really flourishing on the website is the over 50's. It's never too late to form new relationships!

There are only four secrets to having a truly happy relationship:-(enjoy!)

1. It is important to find a person who cooks and cleans.
2. It is important to find a person that makes good money.
3. It is important to find a person who is sensitive to your sexual needs.
4. It is important that these three people never meet!

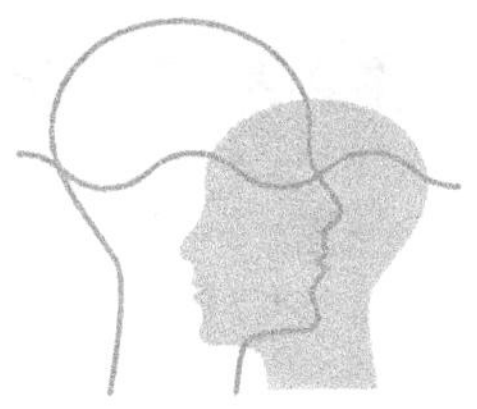

11

Communicating with Others

Communication is so important in any kind of relationship – with a partner, work colleagues, family members, in business dealings, giving a speech. Over the years I have helped many people in my training programs, to strengthen their communication skills. The section, later in this chapter, on *'Responding Decisively'* gives very practical suggestions on how turn a 'yes' answer into 'no' answer, when you really mean 'no'.

<u>The 6 Keys to Effective Communication.</u>

1. Listen with your heart as well as your mind.
2. Don't assume
3. Clarify
4. Don't think – Listen
5. Talk *'with'* not *'at'* the other person
6. Be open-minded and straight forward

<u>Dealing with Problems.</u>

When you want to discuss a problem, choose a time when both parties can give their attention and have the time to talk.

1. **Describe the problem** as you see it. Be brief and speak calmly. Use "I" messages.

    "I feel……….. when…….(describe the problem)." or "When…(Problem)…I feel……..". If you begin your talk with "You ……." it causes the other person to get defensive and nothing gets resolved.

2. **Active listening**. Listen to what the problem is for the other person. Don't judge. Acknowledge their feelings. Repeat if necessary, how it is for you.

3. **Brainstorm solutions**. What can **we** do about it? Listen to the other person. Don't make judgements at this stage. Attack the problem, **not** the person. Be prepared to negotiate the best solution for both of you.

4. **Trial the solution** for a fixed time.

5. **Evaluate**. Is it working? Are any changes needed?

Keep calm, take slow deep breaths when necessary. If things get tense and the discussion is getting off-track, say "This is not working out at the moment. Let's resume when we both feel calmer." ……. words to that effect. Nothing is resolved when people get angry.

Because we are not taught how to listen properly, poor listening skills are the cause of many communication problems. You will find the following pointers helpful.

<u>Do's</u> Of Active Listening.

- Let others finish what they are saying without interrupting them.
- Ask questions if you are confused.
- Pay attention to what others are saying and keep comfortable eye contact.
- Remain open-minded and ready to revise your opinion.
- Use feedback and paraphrasing skills, eg "So what you saying is .. (brief overview)
- Pay attention to non-verbal signals such as the speaker's body language.

<u>Don'ts</u> Of Active Listening.

- Don't rehearse what you are going to say next, while the other person is talking.
- Don't interrupt.
- Don't become defensive.
- Don't change the focus to yourself.
- Don't discount the speaker's reactions as irrelevant or inappropriate.
- Don't judge the rightness or wrongness of the speaker's point of view until you have all the facts.
- Don't solve the problem prematurely.
- Don't say – "I know exactly how you feel." No one knows *exactly* how another person feels.

I hope you find some of these tips helpful. We all have our weaknesses when it comes to using listening skills. Perhaps you could tick the ones you handle well and note the ones you need to fine-tune. Good luck.

Responding Decisively.

Have you said **"Yes"** to someone's request, when you really wanted to say **"No"?** How did that leave you feeling – annoyed, angry, powerless, depressed? Perhaps you don't want to 'rock the boat' or there is a feeling of guilt that you are letting the other person down, or you may be afraid of rejection, or seem selfish, or being put down by the other person if you said 'no'.

Be aware of when you are asked something like – *"What are you doing next Thursday?"* If you say, *"Nothing"* you could be setting yourself up to give a *"Yes"* but I really mean *"No'.* answer. I think many of us have been caught out by that at some time. Your first response could be – *"What's happening on Thursday?"* giving you time to prepare a response. If the request is something that you could do, your *'yes'* response will be genuine. If the request is one that is inconvenient for you, then you have the opportunity to say – *"Unfortunately, I've got something else on that day. Sorry I can't help you."* – words to that effect. You do not actually have to use the word 'no' in your response. The best way to respond more decisively is to practise this technique on simple requests at first.

When you are trying to stick with your 'financial diet' and a friend invites you to go to a concert or something that is expensive for you, what you could say is, *"I'd love to go, but at the moment it is not a priority in my budget and I can't do everything that comes up. Hopefully next time."* Or words to that effect. Again, you don't have to use "no".

If you are feeling pressured in the workplace to do more than your fair share of the workload, could it be that you are saying 'yes' to extra duties when you need to be saying 'no'? Next time you are asked to take on extra work that you know is going to put more pressure on you, you could say something like — *"When do you need this done by, as I am very busy working on this other task. Do you want me to do the new task in place of the present one?"* or *"Because this project is a priority, I would not be able to give this extra task the time it requires."* As mentioned previously, word your response so that you don't have to use the 'no' word.

People at my retirement life planning seminars over the past few years, have shared some interesting stories with me, where saying 'yes' but really wanting to say 'no' can lead to problems. When some couples retire, and decide to buy a motor-home to travel around the country, it is a decision that both people agree on and are excited about their new adventure and had a wonderful trip.

I've met other couples where the husband was keen to buy the motor-home and the wife wasn't, but said 'yes' to keep the peace. Their trip didn't always go well. In fact, some couples part ways during the trip around the country and the wife has hopped on a plane and flown back home because she couldn't handle it anymore. There is a large town in far north Queensland that has a successful business, transporting motor homes back south. Sometimes poor communication skills come to a head, when you are sitting side by side for hours on end as you travel endless kilometres.

A better option would have been for the wife to suggest they rent a motor-home for a few weeks and see how that worked, before they committed to a large expense and a long trip, especially if they haven't done it before. This way she's not actually saying 'No' but offering an alternative which makes sense.

A <u>money-saving tip</u> here is:-If you are keen to buy a motor-home, check out the ones that have been used (or hardly used in some cases!) rather than buying a new one and save your money for the fuel on the big trip.

Sometimes people have unrealistic expectations of others and can put pressure on that person, to carry out a task they aren't competent in carrying out. For example, you may belong to a committee that is organising a large function and a committee member who originally offered to be the co-ordinator, says that she can't do it now. She suggests that you could do it. Even though you are happy to be part of the team, the thought of co-ordinating the whole event is something you feel very inexperienced to do. If you say 'yes' but feel pressured to live up to someone else's expectations, that can be stressful. You could say something like, "Thank you for considering me for this role, but at this point of time I have some personal commitments that take priority. I am happy to take on one of the smaller tasks as the event draws closer." That way you don't have to say 'no'.

Another issue that has surfaced a number of times at the retirement life planning seminars is to do with **minding the grandchildren.** At the beginning of the seminar I ask people what are they most looking forward in retirement and so often they say *'freedom'*. Freedom to do some of the things they have put on hold till they retire, like travel, doing what they want when they want, not answering to a boss. But for some retirees, things don't always work out how they thought.

One couple came up to speak with me after one seminar, to share their story. The husband had been retired for a few years and he and his wife had talked about now being able to go on longer caravan trips than during his work life and see more of Australia. However, his wife can't say 'no' to always being available for minding the grandchildren, so they haven't been away in their caravan. So much for having freedom to do their own thing.

Those of us with grandchildren do love to spend time with them, but I think it is important to weigh up the time you would like to do the things that give you pleasure and the time you can be available to help out with your grandchildren. It is different for everyone. Some people are happy to be available whenever they are asked; others are available at different times.

A couple of my friends who play golf twice a week, have set those boundaries in place with their families. On the days they are not available, their children make other arrangements. When you are going away on a trip, give plenty of notice so that other arrangements can be made for the grandchildren.

When we had small children, we were a long way from our families and I was always able to find carers, whom I paid to mind our children when I was working. When old enough, they went to pre-school. Two of our daughters and their families live in different parts of the country and have also managed with organizing sitters for their children before they started school, when they needed to. We love to visit our daughters when we can and love spending time with our four grandchildren.

I do think that it is important that our children have back-up sitters they can turn to when grandparents get sick or want to travel. What starts out as a great idea – spending time with your grandchildren, can become stressful and tiring if you are missing out on some 'me' time which you deserve in retirement, to enjoy doing some of your own interests.

It gets back to how to say 'no' when you don't actually want to use that word. If you keep saying 'yes', your son/daughter could presume that you don't have any other commitments. I think it is important to set some boundaries early on. Decide which activities mean a lot to you and that you deserve to make time to do them.

Do you have any trips coming up during the year that you want to do? In most instances your children will respect that you need time to do your own thing and it gives them time to organise other minding arrangements.

The happiest arrangements seem to be when the grandparents feel that they can have a say about their availability and reach a compromise.

The secret is to replace the 'No' word with other words, as I have suggested, to make it less stressful to deal with a situation that doesn't suit you.

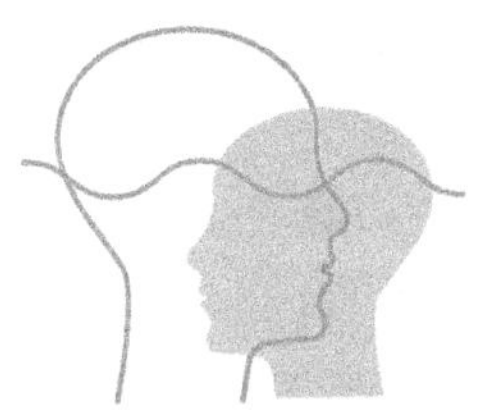

12

Are You Connected or Disconnected?

No, I'm not talking about the internet. I'm talking about the many different ways in our daily lives that we are either connected or disconnected to the people in our lives, responsibilities, work, our values, technology. Let me give you some examples:-

<u>You are connected when you:-</u>

- Spend some time on the computer, but know when to turn it off to do other things like get up and move around – going outside, chatting with others face-to-face.
- Balancing your mode of conversation between written & personal interaction.
- Enjoy regular outdoor activities. A daily 30 minute walk is great for your mental and physical health.
- Taking the time to listen to others and what they are really saying.

- Share regular meals with family members with TV turned off.
- Turn mobile phone off when eating out, to properly enjoy the company of others.
- Turn mobile phone off when attending seminars or meetings, to be properly involved.
- When making presentations, being more focussed on interacting with your audience than putting the main focus on the power point slides.
- Living in the 'now' rather than dwelling on the past or waiting for the future.

You are disconnected when you:-

- Flick emails to work colleagues just nearby, instead of face-to-face contact.
- Constantly checking your mobile phone.
- Spend more time 'chatting' on the internet than chatting in person.
- Spend more time indoors than outdoors.
- Spend too much time thinking of the past or future and not being in the present.
- Feel more connected to the workplace and then 'switch-off' when you get home, preferring to watch TV or go on the computer, rather than engaging in conversation with family members.
- In a presentation, putting your focus on your slide show rather than your audience.

Do a checklist of the two sections. What can you change so that you enhance the quality of your life? Human beings are meant to be social creatures. Having regular conversations face-to-face and interacting socially, benefits our health. There is a growing concern that more and more people, especially the younger generation, are becoming addicted to technology communication. It is here to stay and has many benefits. However, are we becoming more committed to techno relationships than real-life ones? We need to be mindful of the importance of personal interaction and maintaining our social face-to-face communication skills.

The results of a recent 'Essential Report' found that 31% of people regularly check work emails out of hours, 30% on weekends and 21% on holidays. 14% admitted to checking their mobile ph while driving. It was found that 18% of 18-24 year olds get anxious if they don't check text messages every 15 minutes.

A mild addiction to the internet and mobile phone can turn into a serious addiction. Realising that text messages and emails and Facebook are not urgent forms of communication, means that we should be able to 'switch off' from constantly checking them and focus more on giving our attention to the people we are with and also practise safe driving.

I think it is important to set boundaries for how much time, children can use computer games, mobiles, etc. Habits form early in life – much easier than trying to change them later. Having at least a couple of meal times a week with no TV and engaging in conversation around the dinner table, is so valuable for the health of any kind of relationship.

When you speak face-to-face, there is a better understanding of what the communication taking place, is really all about. The tone of your voice and your body language give a good indication of where you are coming from. This can help to avoid the misunderstandings that can occur with text messages. Because the true emotional state of the person texting, does not always come through and things can be misinterpreted. Even though texting is convenient, if emotional issues are involved, a phone call or better still, meeting face-to-face can be more effective. I find it disturbing to hear that people break up relationships or are told they have lost their job via text messages. How impersonal! This can be so devastating for the person receiving the text, much more than if they had been told face-to-face.

> **Every so often, unplug the gadgets and plug into some real communication.**

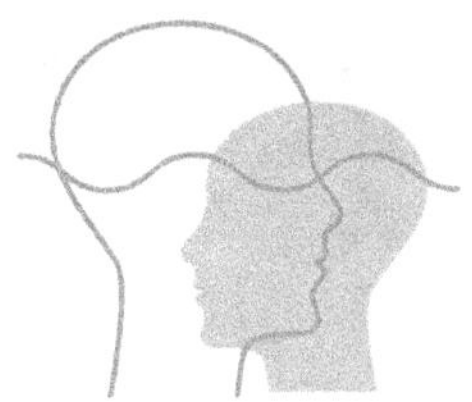

13

The Financial Diet

Since the global financial crisis twelve years ago and now more economic unrest, many people are experiencing uncertain times. This chapter will give you useful tips on how some financial dieting can benefit you. It's easy to get caught up worrying about your super funds and reading negative comments in the media. We are a lot better off than some countries.

Rather than constantly worrying about money, which can easily lead to stress, ill-health and depression, let's look at how to balance saving and spending, so that we can enjoy the freedom that life after full-time work brings. The superannuation industry group ASFA, says that a comfortable retirement will cost the average Australian couple $55,000 a year, a 'modest' lifestyle will cost a couple $31,700 and a single person will need $22,000.

Perhaps the first question to ask yourself is: ***"What is the role of money in my life?"***

Use the following checklist to identify what money means to you:-

- Financial peace of mind
- Financial freedom
- A comfortable lifestyle
- Travelling to interesting new places
- Making a difference to the lives of others
- Professional development
- Investments
- Happiness
- Personal Status
- Fun & adventure

Start a **MONEY DIET** to maintain a sense of control over your life and spending habits. Look at how you can save money on a daily/weekly basis. Make time to shop around for the best deals, whether it's food shopping or larger items.

You may need to change your spending habits and set a realistic budget. You need to ensure that your estate planning is in place, such as wills and power of attorney. Pay off your credit card. If you don't have the money, don't buy it. How often have I heard stories of people who spend up big on motor homes, sailing boats, four-wheel drives, and then regret it. Hire or rent, before you commit to big expenses, especially if it is a new venture – try before you buy. There are some great buys out there, for pre-owned motor-homes that may have only been used a couple of times and you can save quite a lot, instead of purchasing a brand new one. You don't want to chew up your assets and then suffer the consequences of living on less.

Our life can be rich in different ways without spending money all the time. Simple things like eating out less and having more picnics and home entertaining, with everyone contributing, can be fun and you are still socialising, while saving money. Walking, cycling, swimming, are some activities that keep us fit, get us out into nature, mixing with others and cost very little. I think it's important to not deprive yourself of the smaller pleasures that make life happy, like buying a bunch of flowers each week to enhance your living space or going out for coffee with a friends once a week. It's the large expenses we need to trim back.

Spending money on material things all the time, won't relieve boredom. Like children who gets lots of toys and games for Christmas and after a while, they become bored, complaining of nothing to do. A sense of purpose delivers a feeling of achievement and fulfilment; waking up each morning, thinking of the things you want to do that makes you feel like you are really living, which doesn't have to be dependent on having lots of money.

John's story – Retirement is not just about money.

"Five years ago I retired at age 58, as I'd had enough of the daily grind and the routine of battling the traffic, morning and evening. Being blessed with a "comfortable" position financially with my superannuation, chasing that next dollar was not one of my goals.

My wife and I had the obligatory post retirement vacation and a few caravan trips but then a year on, I started to miss the social contact and professional networking that my full time employment provided. I sought casual consulting work in the same field in which I had previously spent 40 years. The shock of getting back into the "cut and thrust" of work that previously filled my life, made me question just why I was back into it. I was torn between the renewed contact with my profession and the long held desire to cut loose. But the fact that it was casual employment taking up no more than around 20% of my time, meant that I could return to "retirement" frequently.

I've taken the approach that at any time, I can walk away from my casual employment if I wish. Such freedom! But in the back of my mind, I still have that niggling worry that I would miss the Industry "chatter", the social contact and the meeting of new people with common professional interests, that my casual employment has provided. However, this is changing gradually as I become more involved in volunteering my time to local community activities. This is providing new social contacts and a satisfying sense of giving something back to the community.

*About 12 months ago I started attending a local **men's shed,** initially for the social benefits, but now I see the need to encourage other guys and to provide social contacts for them. The men's shed concept in my view, is a very valuable addition to the overall retirement experience for many of us guys who have spent so much of our lives, being defined by what we did. Thus the more I get involved the more I see opportunities to help others which I have found to be very rewarding.*

So I have ended up being quite busy in retirement which is a common "complaint" of many retirees, but a good one. My wife and I have still found time to do some overseas travel and we have a small van for local getaways on the odd occasion.

While we are both blessed with fairly good health presently, ageing and health issues sit in the back of my mind. But as you say, there is no point concentrating on the downside of getting old. So we endeavour to get adequate physical exercise and eat healthy food and take a positive approach to managing our health.

After I retired from full time work, I reflected on my experience of preparation for retirement and whether I could have improved on the transition, which of course is still a work in progress. For one thing, I could see the crying need for employers to engage presenters like yourself who could take intending retirees through the type of transition issues you cover in your book, "So What Do We Do Now?". There seems to be a real lack of this sort of thing. As a consequence many people go through the experiences you describe in your book, being poorly equipped to manage them. In talking to colleagues still in the full time workforce contemplating retirement, I'm starting to get feedback that a number of employers are now taking a more holistic approach with pre-retirees, in helping them think about their future outside of their current employment. This is very heartening to hear.

I agree when you point out, that there has previously been (and still is) so much emphasis on financial security — as if that is all that counts. While a reasonable amount of financial security going into retirement is necessary, in these days of a rapidly rising cost of living, money alone simply does not bring contentment in my view.

I think John's story highlights that money is only part of life in retirement and as long as you have adequate for your needs, you don't need to keep working just to have more for the sake of it.

When we go away on trips, one thing my husband and I do to cut costs, is take our thermos and stop along the way in parks to have our morning coffee break, instead of cafes. On a recent trip to New Zealand where we travelled by car around the North island for three weeks, we saved around $200 by organising our own coffee break each day. When travelling by car, we also find it more relaxing to pull up at a scenic spot and have a chance to stretch the legs, breathe in some fresh air and feel refreshed for the next stage of the trip. If we had the occasional wet day, we went to a café. The money we saved, covered the cost of two night's accommodation.

Prioritise your **NEEDS v WANTS**. People have tightened their belts since the global financial crisis in 2008 and now again with the world economic downturn. We have to weigh up whether we can really afford, in the long-term, some of the things we want, but perhaps don't really need.

After one seminar, a woman in her 60's came up to me and said that she had often talked about buying a kayak, once she retired and had more time. She was now retired but she kept putting it off and felt she shouldn't be spending her money on non-essentials. I made her re-think her priorities and putting things on hold until 'later' when it may be too late. She said, *"I am going to buy the kayak tomorrow!"* A few weeks later I received an email from her, saying that it was the best decision she'd ever made!

At first I felt unsure about down-sizing to a duplex five years ago, when we did a return sea-change to where we had lived 20 years earlier. At first, I still wanted the bigger home, but now I enjoy living in our smaller home and the thing I really love is, having less housework – a big plus! As we get older, it becomes a time in our lives to let go of accumulating more material things, de-cluttering and enjoying a simpler lifestyle. Especially now, that in retirement we have the time to go on trips. Some retirees may have the money to go on regular overseas trips. Some retirees may have the money for shorter trips closer to home. There are many great travel options available. Find one to suit your budget and still have a great time.

Review your **VALUES – What is important in my life?** Which areas of your life are you sacrificing or jeopardising by focusing too much on material goals? In the long run will it be worth it. Money issues can colour our thinking about what is important in our lives. Regular social contacts, a sense of community, helping others, can give our lives meaning and take our focus off money issues, especially during financial downturns. The right values are the foundations of a rich and fulfilling life.

I was told this story by a friend at tennis: She knew of a couple in her former rural community who were very wealthy. Even though the husband was a millionaire, he was very mean with his money. He had to go into hospital for major heart surgery which involved getting a heart transplant. His wife visited him every day and was very caring. While still in hospital, he told her, that when he was better, he would take her on an overseas trip and they would also buy a caravan and see more of Australia. She was quite thrilled about the promise and the fact that, he had a change of attitude to money and was now prepared to spend some of it to enjoy life.

However, during his recovery time back at home, he slid back into his old money attitudes and didn't keep his promise. His wife was hurt, let-down and very disappointed in her husband's obsession with not using some of his wealth to enjoy life, especially after his major operation. She decided that she no longer wanted to live under the same roof as him. They didn't divorce but she bought a home in another town where she settled. If he wants to see her, he has to go to the next town to visit her. She has started to make her own life.

Now a quite different story - I read that a millionaire in Vienna, Austria, gave away his fortune of **$5 million** and also his personal possessions to charities, because his wealth *"never made me happy"*. How many times do we hear that money doesn't buy happiness? I firmly believe that valuing our health and relationships will give us a richer life, instead of worrying about money, which can lead to ill-health. Research is showing that some of the happiest places in the world are where people enjoy a strong community spirit and feel needed and valued.

Look into **LIFE PLANNING** – It is so important to think carefully about both financial planning and life planning. With the economic downturns we have experienced over the past four years in particular, many people who had thought of retiring are continuing to work, to build up their nest-egg. You need to ask yourself, *"How much is enough?"*

There are people out there, putting off their retirement till some time down the track, focusing just on the money issues and not really having given any thought to how they are going to spend their time in retirement. If you want to keep working longer because you love what you do, that's great. If you don't like your work and are getting tired, but keep pushing yourself to earn extra money, with no clear plan of how you are going to live in retirement, then you may have a problem. Would you rather be rich or live a rich life? Creating a *'rich'* life will give you the tools to take your mind off worrying constantly about money, and see with fresh eyes, how to live a confident, happy life, that is not just ruled by money issues. What is wealth without health?

Some people combine the travel with part-time work. I met a **retired dentist** and his wife a couple of years ago, when they were passing through our coastal town, on their caravan trip around the country. They had been on the road for a few months and really enjoying their travels. What helped, he said, was that every so often, when they felt like a longer break, the retired dentist would call on the local dentist in the town and ask if he needed some extra help in his dental surgery. Often the local dentist would jump at the offer. It became a win-win for both. The local dentist could catch up on a back-log of work and have some extra time off. The retired dentist got the opportunity to use his skills and earn some extra money to keep financing their trip. And his wife got some time to do her own thing. When the temporary work was complete, they continued their journey. I know of other people who get involved in seasonal work on their travels, like fruit picking to boost their funds.

The more you develop a life plan that includes activities that you want to enjoy, the easier it is to develop a financial plan that will support what you can do. It's important to think of the activities you want to be involved in on a regular basis when you are home and what kind of holidays you can afford and how often you can get away. What are the costs involved to play golf every week? How often can you afford to go out to dinner? There are many questions to ask yourself and discuss with your partner and financial advisor, so that your spending pattern will stretch over a number of years. If you rush into a couple of big overseas trips early in your retirement and then find that you have over-spent too quickly, it will limit what you can do down the track.

At the many seminars at which I have presented on the life planning side of retirement, I have found time and time again, that many pre-retirees and those already retired, were focusing too much on money issues - worrying about not having enough, scared of spending it, or at the other extreme, spending on large items and then regretting it. Now it is even more crucial, in these uncertain times, to look at how to **turn fear into hope**, to survive the financial roller-coaster ride into retirement.

<u>Some words of wisdom from the **Dalai Lama**:-</u> When asked what surprised him most about humanity, the Dalai Lama answered:– *"Man. Because he sacrifices his health in order to make money. Then he spends money in order to recuperate his health. And then he is so anxious about the future that he does not enjoy the present, the result being that he does not live in the present or in the future. He lives as if he is never going to die, and then he dies as if he has never lived."*

Start **NOW** to do some of the things you want to do in retirement – test the waters. This way you are starting to create a more realistic lifestyle plan and also developing a more realistic financial plan, so that you don't put off your retirement any longer than you need to. Good financial advice can help you to enjoy the fruits of your labour and still have enough money put away, so that you can spend time doing the things you enjoy without spending all your money.

Time is free, but it is priceless.
You can't own it, but you can use it.
You can't keep it, but you can spend it.
Once you've lost it, you can never get it back.

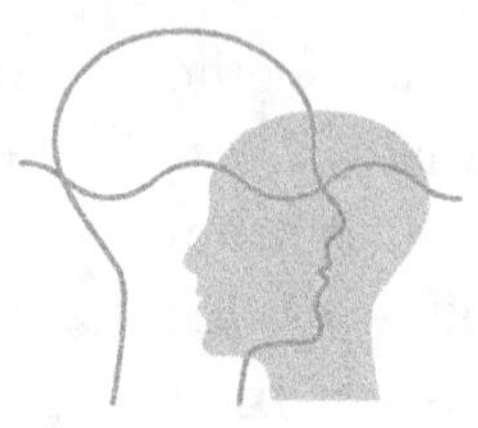

14

Life is a Balancing Act

Some people have been so taken up with their work life, that other areas of their life have had a low priority. So when they finally finish full-time work, it's like their life can suddenly come to a standstill. Start now, to make time for other things in your life besides work, so that when you stop working one day down the track, you already have other interests to fill your days.

A few years ago, I ran a number of workshops on **'Work/Life Balance'** for various companies on the importance of creating a balance in the 6 key areas of life:-

- Our work life - live to work or work to live
- Our relationships – family, partners, community
- Our health – mental, physical and emotional
- Our leisure time – pursuing interests that we enjoy

- Our finances - realistic budgeting
- Our goals – future plans

It gave the participants a wake-up call on how imbalanced our lives can get, when we put our main focus on just one of the six areas – namely work. It is important to ask yourself ***"Am I living to work, or working to live?"***

<u>Stop – Look –Listen</u>

No, I'm not talking about stopping at the road traffic lights. But then, I could quite easily make an analogy to our own internal 'traffic lights'.

The **orange** light comes on when we are rushing around too much and getting stressed. It is warning us that it's time to slow down in our lives. But do we always listen? If we ignore the orange light and don't see the **stop** light coming, it's a bit like the traffic cop suddenly coming up behind and pulling you over, making you stop.

The **'internal' stop sign** can be something like a bad bout of the flu, a sprained ankle, a back injury, etc, something that leaves us with no choice, but to stop and rest. At first this can be stressful, feeling guilty about not carrying out your normal routine. However, when you accept the situation and stop fighting it, this can end up being quite a blessing in disguise.

When we tune into our own traffic lights and listen to the signals to slow down, we can get into the habit of slowing down each day, rather than **'crash'** because we haven't listened to our body signals. Have a break from the computer and any activities that can cause a build up of stress. Get outside every so often – sit in the sun, go for a walk – switch off the busy mind and instead focus on breathing in the fresh air, looking at the clouds, trees, water, whatever – just relaxing and letting go of thinking about problems. Curling up and reading a good book is another way to *'let go'*.

Sometimes we need to put the brakes on, slow down and recharge the batteries. Otherwise we can miss those magic moments in life that happen spontaneously and bring us a feeling of happiness that money can't buy.

When the **green light** comes on, it is a sign to move forward with hope, feel more balanced and have faith that you don't have to stress about how things are going and not needing to control the outcome.

<u>So remember:-</u>

Orange light – slow down
Red light – stop and recharge the batteries, relax
Green light – Move forward again, but feeling more balanced and less stressed.

Have a safe and happy trip!

Since writing my first book and presenting at many seminars over the past twenty years on life planning, I have realised just how important it is to take work/life balance seriously from early on in your working life. Then, when the time comes to deal with life's changes, the fear of *"What will I do all day?"* will be reduced significantly and the possibility of depression diminished, because work hasn't been your only focus.

Here is a **story** I came across a few years ago and I think is *'food for thought'*.

A fisherman was sitting on the beach near the water's edge. A single fishing rod was planted in the sand next to him. Along came a businessman on vacation.

"Why don't you have two poles so you can catch more fish?" he asked the fisherman.

"Then what would I do?" *"Then you could use the extra money to buy a boat, get nets and a crew and catch even more fish."* replied the businessman.

"Then what would I do?" *"Then,"* said the businessman, *"you could move up to a fleet of large ships, go wholesale and become very rich."*

"Then what would I do?" **"Then you can do whatever you want!"** shouted the exasperated businessman, to which the fisherman replied, **"I am."**

This story can give us a reality check. Is all the extra work we can end up doing, improving the quality of our life?

A survey taken a few years ago, found that 42% of full-time workers found it difficult to disconnect from work when they got home; 40% of families believed they had no choice in balancing work/home life; workers' compensation claims for stress-related illnesses had increased 400% in the last 10 years!

It is important to *'switch-off'* from work when you get home, but that doesn't mean to *'switch-on'* the TV as soon as you get home and not interacting with your family and partner. In the longer daylight hours of summer, it is an ideal time to spend some time outside after work, going for walks, do some gardening, especially if you have a sedentary indoor job and may spend a lot of time in front of the computer.

It is important to schedule time to unwind and relax. This gives you the chance to collect your thoughts. Often busy people don't stop to focus on whether all their energy is being used up in an area, that ultimately isn't that important to them. Putting on some relaxing music helps, as does going for a relaxing walk, that gives you enough time to unwind and de-clutter your busy mind.

Just as we know that we need a balanced diet to keep healthy, we also need a balanced life style to stay mentally and physically fit. Regular walks are important if you have a sedentary job.

Most of us know that to become successful, we need an education and training in learning new skills. Did you know that enjoying life is also a learned behaviour? Training yourself to enjoy life is as important as training yourself to achieve. The more we develop and practice the skills to enjoy life, the happier and more fulfilling our life can become. This will involve changing some old thought patterns that can be holding us back from enjoying life, as mentioned earlier. It also means giving yourself permission to take time out of your busy schedule to start making some changes.

Is work consuming a large chunk of your time, with only a small amount left over for your personal life? Are you living to work or are you working to live? How can you bring the ratio closer to 50/50 to create a better work/life balance? Can you learn to make-do, with the accumulation of less material things, which seems to be a major reason for people over-working and getting stressed?

The following story (author unknown) is cleverly written and appropriate to this chapter.

The Professor and the Jar – A professor stood before his philosophy class and had some items in front of him. He picked up a very large empty jar and proceeded to fill it with golf balls. He then asked the students if the jar was full. They agreed that it was.

Then the professor picked up a box of pebbles and poured them into the jar. He shook the jar lightly and the pebbles rolled into the open areas between the golf balls. He then asked the students again if the jar was full. They agreed that it was.

Next the professor picked up a box of sand and poured it into the jar. Of course the sand filled up the remaining space. He asked once more if the jar was full. The students responded with an unanimous "Yes!"

The professor then produced two cups of coffee from under the table and poured the entire contents into the jar, effectively filling the spaces between the grains of sand.

"Now," said the professor, as the laughter subsided, "I want you to recognise that this jar represents your life. The **golf balls** are the important things – your family, your health, your friends and your favourite passions – things that if everything else was lost and only they remained, your life would still be full. The **pebbles** are the other things that matter like your job, your house, your car. The **sand** is everything else – the small stuff."

"If you put the sand into the jar first," he continued, "there is no room for the pebbles or the golf balls. The same goes for life. If you spend all your time and energy on the small stuff, you will never have room for the things that are important to you. Pay attention to the things that are critical to your happiness. Play with your children. Take time to get medical checkups. Take your partner out to dinner. Take time to relax.

How often do you need to clean the house? How much TV do you watch? Take care of the golf balls first, the things that really matter. **Set your priorities.** The rest is just sand.

Then one of the students raised her hand and inquired what the coffee represented. The professor smiled. "I'm glad you asked. It just goes to show you that no matter how full your life may seem, there is always room for a cup of coffee with a friend."

I have remembered that interesting analogy of the golf balls, pebbles and sand, as a way to keep a check on what is important, to keep a balance in my own life. I hope it helps you too.

Stop gulping life down. Sip it like a fine wine, savouring every drop. It's so important to enjoy life in the present, capturing the simple joys of everyday life, instead of putting it on hold till 'later'.

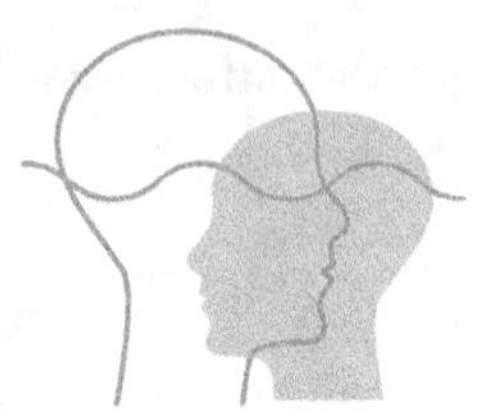

15

Lighten The Load

Do you find yourself, whether you are working or retired, pulled in too many different directions, trying to do too many things and trying to please too many people? Is this draining your energy, causing you stress and depriving you of time you would like to spend on your interests? Then it's time to get back in the driver's seat and enjoy the journey of your life, with a better balance of work, health, family, responsibilities, social life, and more time to do the things that give you joy.

To set some boundaries, go through this questionnaire.

1. What makes you feel happy and energised?
2. Which people in your life make you feel good?

3. What is draining your energy?
4. How important is this in the big picture/
5. What would you like to spend more/less time on?
6. What is stopping you at this point in time?
7. What can you do differently?
8. What will it take?

A few years ago when I ran "Work/Life Balance" workshops, I would give this questionnaire to the participants. It helped them to develop a greater awareness of what to change, in order to improve their quality of life, and to realise that it wasn't selfish to address some of their own needs. However, the challenge was to go back to their busy work life and not falling into the trap of saying – *"Sounds a great idea, but I'm too busy to put it into practice."* Nothing changes if we don't make a commitment, to put in the time and effort to create a more balanced life style. So easy for work to take over your life!

After one of my life planning presentations, a man who had been retired for 5 years came up to me and said that, some of the things he thought were so important before he retired, hadn't been that important in the big picture. He realised now that he had wasted precious time and energy that he could have spent on other more meaningful things in his life. And guess what? None of us are indispensible. Life goes on and people cope without us.

If you are telling yourself that you are too busy and haven't the time to do this life-changing questionnaire, you may be caught up in some activities that really are draining your time and energy. Five years down the track you may look back and wish that you had prioritised things differently.

Listen to your self-talk and notice if you tend to say *'should'* or *'could'*. When we say *'should'* a lot it implies a sense of duty, guilt, stress, obligation. When we turn the *'should'* into *'could'* it implies choices, changes, flexibility, less stress.

Another way to *'lighten the load'* in our daily lives is to do with our mindset. Unrealistic expectations about people, events, money, can leave us feeling disappointed, angry, resentful, depressed. It can mean things like – looking for the perfect relationship, expecting a promotion and it doesn't happen, expecting people to treat you a certain way, etc. Unrealistic expectations lead to disappointment and anger because things didn't turn out the way we thought they 'should'. We miss the opportunity to see what is good in our life and the habitual negative thinking of unrealistic expectations, drains our physical and mental energy.

Hanging onto the vision of how something *'should'* be, can stop you seeing the new opportunities coming into your life, that can actually be better for you. Just by accepting that we are all different and doing the best we can and looking for the good in others, can improve the quality of our own lives and lighten the load.

Keep saying, **"Something better is coming into my life."**

Daily appreciation of the good in our lives dissolves the feelings of disappointment and negativity that unrealistic expectations create. Being thankful for the good in our lives, grounds us in the present, a glancing back, with thanks for *'what was'* and projecting forward to what *'could be'* – our hopes and dreams. Get into the habit of being thankful for the good things in your life, no matter how small. You will feel less stressed and attract less conflict into your life. We can tend to worry about the things we don't have and take for granted the many things that we are fortunate to have. When you find yourself getting bogged down about an issue that is stressing you, ask yourself – *"In the big picture, how important will this be in a month or a year's time?"*

Why not start a Gratitude Journal in a small notebook, that you can keep next to your bed. Before you go to sleep, write down 5 things that you are thankful for that day, comments like – *"I am thankful for my good health, finding the car keys, living in a peaceful country, loving what I do."* On the days that haven't been that good, read some of the previous pages, to remind yourself of all the good in your life. This lifts your spirits and stops you getting stuck in negative thinking and you sleep better. By thinking more about all the things that are going right in your life and less about all the things that have gone wrong, you will lift your spirits. Instead of dwelling on what's not working, change your thoughts to what you could do, to improve the situation.

It's easy to get caught up in the 'busyness' of our everyday lives. We don't allow ourselves that quiet time to just switch off, retreat and take stock of how our lives are really going. I urge you to make the time, when you are more relaxed, to find a quiet space and take a raincheck on your life, to get a clearer picture of how you can **'lighten the load'**. Then start doing one thing differently and persist for 3 weeks, because that is about how long it takes to create a new habit. What always helps me is to say to myself – *"What is the worst thing that could happen?"* Then get on with it. I have found that when you make that statement and answer it, everything feels more manageable.

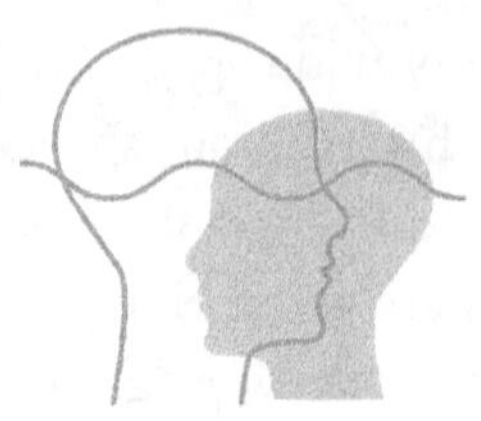

16

Pull All The Weeds Out Now!

After house-sitting for my sister for a few months last year, I returned home at the start of the Spring season, to a well-mown yard and healthy looking plants. However, one thing my husband does not like to do, is the weeding! That has always been my task which fortunately, I enjoy doing. Weeding helps me with two things – defusing any tension I'm feeling, or better still, sparking off a great idea. That is what happened during one of my weeding sessions. As I was madly pulling out the weeds, the thought suddenly came to me, about how we can *pull out the weeds* in our life!

Spring is the season for new life and new growth and by removing the weeds that hinder growth, we give the new, emerging plants the opportunity to grow and blossom.

What is hindering your growth as a person? If we were to remove the *'weeds'* in our lives, the things that hinder our growth and can stop us from reaching our full potential, just imagine what an amazing person you could blossom into!

So where to start? How about weeding out all the *'stuff'* you don't really use in your home:- wardrobes, study, pantry, garage, cupboards, etc. One thing I discovered when I was house-sitting for 4 months, was how much of my *'stuff'* I didn't miss while I was away. Now that I've finished weeding the garden, I'll start weeding out the things I don't use, that are just cluttering up my space. I like the saying **–'When you de-clutter, you make room for new things to come into your life.'**

Is the garden of your life overflowing with too many responsibilities that are draining your energy? Why not weed some of them out and delegate to others. This also means letting go of things being done differently to how you would do it. The upside is, that it gives you the chance to grow and blossom in other areas of your life.

Are there people in your life who are hindering your growth? Can you weed them out and let the right relationships have room to blossom and enhance your life.

Weed out the old, limiting beliefs that can hinder your growth. Focus on nurturing the growth of more positive thoughts that can help you to grow and prosper. Why not start today, by pulling out a couple of *'weeds'* that you no longer want growing in your life. Then each week pull out another one, till you feel new growth and new life emerging.

As you pull the weeds out, you lighten your load. Happy gardening!

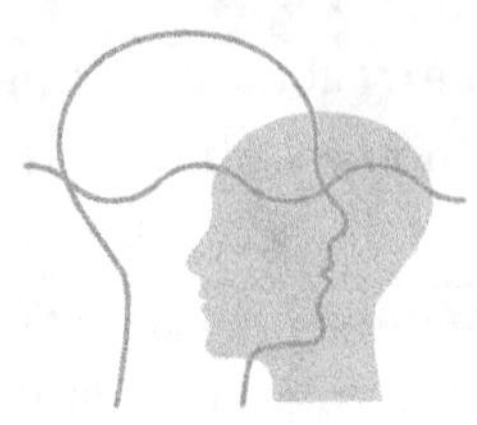

17

Slow Down the Ageing Process

– It's All in The Mind

> *"Age is an issue of mind over matter. If you don't mind, it doesn't matter."* – Mark Twain

Did you know that we have control over how we use our mind? Research shows that our attitude has a strong influence on speeding up or slowing down the ageing process. No matter what our age is at the moment, whether we are in our 20's or 70's, we can learn to control the way we use our mind to keep mentally fit and physically fit.

Our constant thoughts are a self-fulfilling prophecy: Think *'old'* and you feel *'old'*. Think *'young'* and you can feel *'younger'* than your chronological age. ***"Live life, forget your age"*** is a saying that I think is so powerful. In our youth- obsessed western society, girls in their teens worry about getting old. Not a healthy thought to have running around in the mind at such an early age!

As author and poet, Oliver Wendell Holmes once said – ***"To feel seventy years young is far more cheerful than to feel forty years old."***

"Think young and do what you love." This is the philosophy of a friend of ours, who is the leader of a swing band. The swing band is made up of 18 musicians, ranging in age from 26 to 85 years. Our friend says that the mix of ages, keeps the older musicians young at heart. After one concert, I chatted with the group and was amazed when one of the men said he was 85. He looked and acted much younger. Having a purpose and a positive outlook, certainly proved that if we think and feel younger than we are, we can look younger and healthier, so slowing down the ageing process.

I believe that if we have *'fear'* thoughts about ageing, we will age quicker than someone who accepts the ageing process as the natural flow of life and sees new opportunities for continued growth. Research has found that as much as 80% of our physical illnesses can stem from negative thought patterns.

Back in the 1970's Louise Hay wrote her best-selling book – *"You Can Heal Your Body"* in which she discusses the mental patterns that create our physical illnesses. She shows how to create positive thought patterns to heal these illnesses. I have found this book a source of inspiration for many years. For example, with 'ageing problems' Louise Hay says the probable causes are negative thoughts on social beliefs, old thinking, fear of being one's self, rejection of the now. She suggests these new, positive thoughts to replace the old ones – *"I love and accept myself at every age. Each moment in life is perfect."* To make this new thought pattern a habit, it needs to be practised regularly. It takes around 14 daily practices to create a new habit.

I would like to share a **story** with you that highlights how our thought patterns can affect our health. On one of my flights around Australia to present at seminars, I sat next to a 77 year old man. We got into conversation and he told me how he had retired 20 years earlier from a successful real estate business in a rural town. He and his wife relocated to the Gold Coast in Queensland, where they had enjoyed many holidays.

After a couple of years, they decided to try a different kind of business venture and bought a coffee shop. When the contracts had been signed, the wife suddenly decided that she wanted 'out' and returned to their former hometown. They ended up divorcing and he did say the marriage had been shaky and he thought a fresh start in a new place would help. He ended up running the coffee shop for 4 years to get his original investment back. He then invested in another real estate business on the Gold Coast, but that didn't work out and he lost money.

A couple of years after that, he married a second time. And just when he thought that his luck had changed, he was diagnosed with diabetes and soon after with Parkinson's disease! Up until twelve years ago, he had been a healthy person all his life. I was surprised that he didn't have the shakes commonly associated with Parkinson's disease, which he attributed to a new medication he was taking.

Basically his luck changed when he moved from his hometown. Nothing seemed to go right for him in his personal or business life. He felt he'd lost control of his life and regretted leaving his hometown to move to the Gold Coast.

When I returned home from my trip, I looked up diabetes and Parkinson's disease in Louise Hay's book, *"You can Heal Your Body"* and I was amazed to read that both illnesses related to a longing for what might have been and also a need to feel in control. When constant thoughts of regret play on the mind, sickness can develop.

To look after our health, we need to change the thinking patterns that can pull us down, and change them to more positive thought patterns that can lift us up. This is not so easy to do. Old thinking patterns are quite entrenched but with regular practice, we **can** turn around our thinking and lead a healthier, happier life.

Ageing has commonly been associated with the decline of health, memory, looks, abilities. No wonder many people dread the thought of retiring. With millions of baby boomers starting to retire, the face of ageing is starting to change, especially as we are living longer.

Declining **brain function** has been one of the greatest concerns of ageing. However the good news is, that research is showing, that there is **not** a progressive loss of one's thinking abilities. The human brain is continually adapting and rewiring itself in response to new stimuli and new experiences. Research is also finding that age does not affect the rate of learning new information and remembering it. It is also comforting to know, that at least 70% of people who live beyond 85 years won't get Alzheimer's. So we are not 'losing our marbles' as we age!

'Maintain a Healthy Brain'

A recent study in Thailand of women aged 50-60, showed that after 6 months of taking **ginger**, their memory and cognitive function improved. There is growing evidence that ginger has a neuro-protective function which could be helpful for conditions such as Alzheimer's. Add 100 grams of grated ginger to stir-fries to stimulate your brain power. We can all use ginger more often!

A study in USA found that after eating **mashed potatoes**, the subjects' memories improved 32%. Forget the chips. Bring on the mashed potatoes!

Our brain cells can get 'rusty' from lack of use. When you retire and have a lot more time to fill in, you can <u>boost your brain and memory</u> by doing things like:- crosswords, jigsaws, learning a new language or a musical instrument. Just as we exercise the body, we also need to exercise the brain to keep it active. ***'Use it'*** **or** ***'Lose it.'***

Things that can lead to mental decline and hasten the ageing process are - stress, poor nutrition, lack of sleep, worry, anger, too much caffeine and alcohol. They all affect our ability to think and remember clearly and can lead to mental decline.

Brain Fitness Tips

- A <u>good night's sleep</u> regenerates the brain.
- <u>Positive thoughts</u>, including daily gratitude for the good in your life, reduces stress and strengthens the immune system. We think more clearly when we aren't stressed.
- <u>A daily walk</u> and focussed breathing, rejuvenates the brain. Walking is especially good for the brain, because it increases blood circulation and the oxygen and glucose that reach your brain. Maybe this is why walking 'clears your head' and helps you think better. Walk with a friend.
- <u>Eating well</u> - especially fresh fruit and vegetables. **Bananas** are full of potassium which is great for mental alertness, helps with sleep and is helpful for headaches. If I am having trouble sleeping, I get up and eat a banana. In a new study, researchers found that **consuming cocoa** every day improves memory loss. As rich dark chocolate is made up of 70% cocoa, I like this!!

- Drinking moderately, laughing more, enjoying friendships and the simple pleasures of life each day, can all help to keep the brain fit and slow down the ageing process.
- Our brain shrink about 10% as we age, but studies show that keeping our brains fit, can slow that down. Eat nuts like walnuts and almonds.

I read an article about Alzheimer's recently that said regular physical activities like walking and swimming can help to slow down the progression of the disease which destroys the brain cells. It also says that if we make physical exercise part of our daily life, we have a good chance of not getting it in the first place.

A recent study looked at the physical activity in Australians over 65. Results showed that 32% did not exercise in the past year, 40% participated in one activity. Of those, 53% only walked.

To make physical exercise a daily habit, is so important for our health, as I have now mentioned a few times (because it is so important!) Keep the body moving and prevent your joints stiffening up, improve circulation, keep the brain fit, keep depression at bay, reduce stress, improve strength, flexibility and balance, slow muscle wasting - the list just goes on.

I read a report of a study that had been undertaken, that demonstrated how ageing can be slowed down, when people don't act their age. During a week's retreat, the subjects of the study – a group of 75yr olds in good health, were encouraged to think, feel and act as if they were 20 years younger. They played music that was popular 20 years earlier. Compared to the control group who acted their age, the make–believe group improved their manual dexterity and their memory became more active and self-sufficient. Before and after photos showed their faces looking younger and fresher. The study showed that positive expectations and beliefs about ageing, help to create a more vital, healthy experience.

How often do we hear — ***"Happiness comes from within."*** ***"Beauty comes from within."*** When you meet someone who is truly happy with their life, their eyes shine and they have a lovely aura about them. You can have all the beauty treatments in the world and the most expensive clothes, but if you are constantly thinking negatively about your life and other people, this will show through.

So if we want to slow down the ageing process, start thinking good thoughts every day and be thankful every day for the good in your life. **Remember, it's all in the mind.**

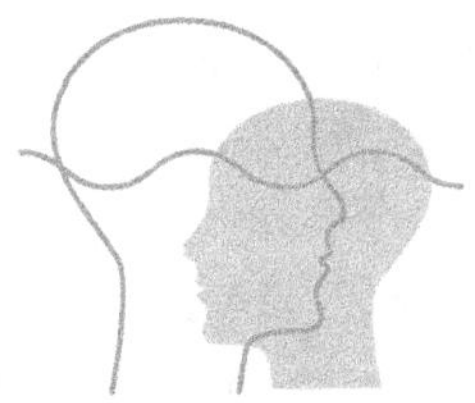

18

Looking Younger Naturally

"*You look great for your age!*" is the best compliment a woman over 50 can receive. One hundred years ago, 50 was old and not many people lived into their 60's. Today, the average life expectancy for women is well into their 80's. Women today are benefiting from advances in health and skin care products, to look younger as they live longer. Women in their 50's and 60's are the Baby Boomers, who are changing all the previous rules about ageing and we are a long way from the finish line!

Meryl Streep, the actress who is in her early 60's, is an inspirational woman who looks great for her age. In a media interview, she talked about her acting career going as well as ever. Streep said, "*It's a miracle that movie roles keep coming. In the past, women my age were absolutely one foot in the old age home. In terms of the work, it gets richer as you get older and you have a bank of experience to draw from."*

Today's baby boomers, especially women, don't feel their age. We still want to look good, but with all the persuasive advertising about cosmetic surgery, promising to make us look *'young forever'* it can lead to women avoiding the reality of ageing, especially physical ageing. The fear thoughts and denial of ageing can actually lead to depression and hasten the ageing process.

Why not accept that our physical features are slowly maturing and get on with living life to the full and stop thinking about ageing, as Meryl Streep is doing so well. We are all getting older, but we don't ever have to think of ourselves as *'old'*. Having the right attitude, as discussed earlier, keeps us feeling younger. Our thoughts create our reality, so rather than focusing on fear thoughts of ageing that can speed up the ageing process, think more about the positives, like, at this stage of our lives we can let go of trying to please other people, just be ourselves, share the wisdom we have gained during our lifetime. If you look in the mirror every day and lament the ageing process, it doesn't make it go away, rather it brings it on faster. Get out there and get involved in meaningful activities that take your mind off ageing.

Ageing is inevitable. From the day we are born to the day we leave this earth, we are **all** ageing. Yet, many people are in denial of this fact. Even young women today worry about ageing and are seeking cosmetic procedures to maintain a 'forever young' appearance. Slowing down the development of ageing skin, is a fine balance between looking great naturally and not overdoing cosmetic procedures.

I was reading a story recently about a 37 year old woman, who had an anti-wrinkle Botox treatment to look younger. She was told that the bruises to her forehead, where she had the injections, would heal in a week and the smoothness would last 3-6 months. Towards the end of the third month, her face was back to its original state. The comment she made was, that she didn't feel any better or any worse about herself. She felt that the benefits were not enough to continue getting Botox. Not to mention the money she would be saving!

According to the Cosmetic Physicians Society of Australasia, Australians spent over $640 million in the past year, on cosmetic treatments, with anti-wrinkle treatments like Botox. Because this treatment is not a 'once off' and needs to be repeated every few months, it can eventually lead to damaged skin, especially if younger people start using it too soon. I have seen 'before and after' photos in magazines, of celebrities who have had Botox treatments. In many cases the original photos, before they started the treatments, are much more flattering than the photos taken a few years later. Botox treatments only temporarily hide the wrinkles and you need ongoing regular treatments to keep 'hiding' them which can actually weakens the facial muscles.

Even if you do have cosmetic procedures, it is vital to take steps on a daily basis to look after your skin and keep it healthy. We age from the inside out, so our emotional well-being and how we look after our bodies, affects our health and skin.

About 25 years ago, I developed an interest in **aromatherapy,** when it was still fairly new in Australia. I was 40 at the time and was keen to look after my skin with natural products. I studied everything I could get my hands on, about **essential oils** and eventually created my own aromatherapy workshops. For a number of years I ran many workshops and shared with others, the wonderful benefits of aromatherapy.

My skin-care workshops were very popular, where I taught women and sometimes men too, how to blend different essential oils to create their own skin creams and other skin-care products. I have used Jojoba Oil for many years as a base for my anti-ageing face oil, to which I add a blend of essential oils like lavender, geranium and frankincense, that have cell-regenerating properties. Rosehip oil and Coconut oil are two other natural oils that have rich antioxidant properties which can help to prevent premature ageing, by delaying wrinkles and sagging skin. Much safer than having Botox treatments.

Much focus is placed on the face ageing, but it is just as important to look after the skin on other parts of your body – like the neck, arms and legs. Often women focus on facial treatments and forget about nourishing the neck, which can be the give-away of ageing skin. Using essential oils blended into a carrier oil like olive oil, makes a wonderful massage oil that can be used on a daily basis, to keep your skin toned up, stimulate circulation, promote elasticity and helps to tighten loose skin and reduce aches in joints.

Steps to Slow Down Skin Ageing:

1. **Eat plenty of antioxidant rich foods**_such as brightly coloured fruit and vegetables. Antioxidants are nutrients (vitamins and minerals) and enzymes (proteins) inside your body that can help to prevent and repair damage to your body's tissue. They do this by slowing down the effect of free radicals which start oxidation. As antioxidants block the damaging effects of free radicals, the antioxidants end up being oxidised. That is why it is important to constantly replenish your intake of antioxidants.

Antioxidant- rich foods, like fresh fruit and vegetables, nuts and grains and fish, can have a positive effect on your skin's health and appearance. **Avocadoes** contain antioxidants that can help protect the skin from premature ageing. It can also be used as an oil. Did you know that **apples** have a very high antioxidant content, so *"An apple a day keeps your skin healthy"* can help us to look younger longer. What a simple and inexpensive way to look after our health and skin! Yet research shows that 46% of Australians only eat an apple once a week.

2. **Vitamins A and C** are thought to be particularly helpful in skin care. They encourage cell and tissue growth which makes them helpful for anti-ageing. These vitamins may also help to reduce wrinkles.

3. **Aloe Vera** is one of the oldest medicinal plants known to man and its incredible effects on the skin were 're-discovered' in the 1970's. It is one of the most powerful antioxidants to occur naturally. Aloe Vera is an excellent skin moisturiser, rejuvenating the skin, hydrating it and increasing its elasticity. Every so often, I take one of the leaves of the Aloe Vera plant growing in our garden, split the leaf open and rub the gel over my face. I leave it on for about 10 minutes and then rinse it off. A simple, natural and inexpensive way to benefit from its cell regenerating properties.

4. Avoid excess sugar. Research shows that a high intake of sugar can cause skin wrinkling.

5. Don't smoke. Free radical production, generated by smoking, ages the skin

6. Avoid prolonged midday sun exposure. Too much sun, fast-forwards ageing

7. Drink up to 2 litres of water a day to keep skin hydrated. Dehydrated skin tends to sag.

8. Get a good night's sleep. Poor sleep can hasten the ageing process.

9. Think more positively and less negatively

10. Smile and be thankful for the good in your life.

As you can see, there are a lot of different ways we can look younger longer – ways that use every day, natural processes that are non-invasive and not expensive. Looking after the whole body – inside and out, having a sound mind, eating well and regular exercise, all work as a team to keep us healthy and looking good.

Make peace with the ageing process: We live in a society that seems to value youth more than valuing ageing. While not easy in our *'youth-obsessed'* world, try and look at life as a series of cycles – each with its own beauties and lessons. Don't buy into the belief that growing older needs to be associated with decline and pity. Take inspiration from the long-living people who have remained purposeful throughout their life and understood that real beauty is found not in how we look, but in who we are.

Following are some stories of people who *'live life and forget their age.'*

- A 98 year old woman who is a marriage celebrant, has no thoughts of stopping yet as she loves meeting people and enjoys what she does!
- A 70 year old female swimming instructor who has coached 40,000 children over 50 years is still going strong despite two bouts of cancer.

- A 94 year old man who belongs to a local swimming club, recently returned from Italy where he competed in the World Masters' Games, winning 4 gold medals, 2 silver medals and one bronze. He started competitive swimming upon his retirement at 80!

- A former surgeon, in his early 70's, uses his skills to perform cleft palate operations in third world countries with Rotary.

- Louise Hay, author of the best-selling book, "You Can Heal Your Life" still travelled the world presenting lectures at 85.

- What about the 100 year old doctor in the USA who **still** practised and credited his happy marriage and love of playing the violin, plus still enjoyed his work, as having kept him healthy.

> *"The secret of life is enjoying the passage of time."*

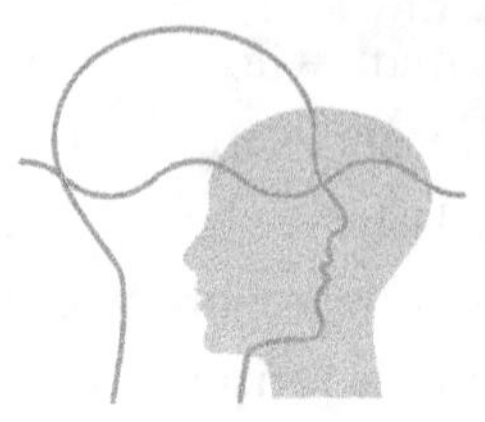

19

The 6 Ingredients to Cook Up A Great Life

"Bask in the rewards of your accomplishments."

The following **6 ingredients** can add flavour to your life whether you are working or have retired. If you don't want your life to get stale, you need to get the right mix of ingredients to create a great recipe for the rest of your life. Too much or too little of an ingredient, can spoil the end result. This final chapter is also a bringing together, of key points that have been covered in other chapters. So what are the six ingredients?

1. **REVIEW**: This is a very important ingredient. What gives meaning to your life? For many years, things like your job and raising a family, give purpose to your life, interspersed with annual holidays and perhaps a hobby or sport. Develop some interests outside of work time, during the years you are employed.

There are many options to give your life meaning. Give yourself time to adjust and re-invent yourself after major life changes. It doesn't happen overnight. It can take on average, five years to create a new way of living in retirement for example. Take into account all the skills, knowledge, experience and wisdom you have developed during your working life, which can now be used to create a purposeful and interesting new life and still go on holidays when you want.

There are so many inspiring stories in the media, of people well into their 80's, who still lead active, healthy and happy lives, because they have a reason to get up in the morning – whether it be still working part-time in a job they love, volunteering, mentoring younger people, learning new things, developing a hobby into a small business. Now that you have the time, explore ways in which you can develop meaning and purpose.

2. **HEALTH**: This is a vital ingredient – the foundation for cooking up a great life. Not just physical, but mental and emotional fitness are so important as well, if we are to lead a healthy life and keep our brains functioning effectively. **Physical fitness** – One of the best things you can do to maintain and improve your health can be something as simple as a daily walk. A regular 2km walk can be a defence against dementia, tones up the physical body and if you can, walk with a friend or in a walking group. The social interaction is also very beneficial for your mental & emotional well being. **Watch your thoughts** – Research in the past few decades has shown that our thoughts impact on our emotions and then on our physical health. 80% of our health problems can be attributed to constant worry and negative thinking. It has been found that people who live to 100, have positive mental attitudes, looking more on the bright side of life, rather than dwelling on what's wrong.

3. **MONEY**:Remember the Abba song – *"Money, money, money, it's a rich man's world"*? But are rich people always happy people? If this is the dominating ingredient in your life, then not a good recipe. Having a lot of money does not always equate with a better quality of life. Worrying constantly about money, hoarding it and not using it to enjoy your life, can affect your health as mentioned in the previous section. Some people worry about never having enough money. But then, how much is enough? That's why it is so important to have a life plan for retirement, to compliment the financial plan. Then you'll have a much better idea how much you will need to finance your activities and be less likely to rush into big expenses that can chew up your assets. It is much better to 'try before you buy' – rent or hire and see how the idea of selling up your home to make a sea change, or buying a motor home works for you.

    How often have I heard people say after having a health crisis, that HEALTH is more important than WEALTH. There is an older man with only one leg, who walks in the park near our place. Whenever I see him as I go walking past, I think to myself that I would rather have my own two legs, than all the money in the world, as I love my walks, bike riding and swimming.

4. **FREEDOM**: In earlier generations, retirement usually meant staying in the family home for the final years of life and winding down. Today, retirees have so many more choices about where to live, travel opportunities, when to actually finish working, to name a few. Sometimes the choices and changes in this new stage of life, can be overwhelming. So often in seminars, pre-retirees tell me the thing they most look forward to is *'freedom'* – to do what they like when they like.

I do think that the more you consider your choices, well before retirement, the less daunting it is. For much of your work life, the routines of everyday life are fairly well set in place. It is easy to say – *"One day.... Later....* talking about the things that you'll do in the future. When you finish full-time work, those former structures and routines will be gone and you will now have a blank page to create the life you want and let go of old habits and commitments that no longer serve you. Retirement can finally be that time in your life to have the freedom to start doing new things, having more time for hobbies, volunteering, family, travel.

Some people embrace this new life and freedom with excitement and anticipation; others with nervousness at the thought of making changes. Sometimes old patterns can be hard to change. Just don't keep putting it off till later, because that can be too late. Is worry about money holding you back from doing something you would now love to do? You can't take it with you when you leave this earth. We have one life so let's make the most of it!

5. **RELATIONSHIPS**: Having friendly associations with others in our lives – family, friends, neighbours, work colleagues. How we relate with others can affect our health and well being. **Communication** is a very important ingredient to add the right mix to the other ingredients, especially when there are money issues to discuss, important choices to make and boundaries to set. If you want some freedom to enjoy your retirement, then you need to communicate your wishes to family members and set some boundaries of your availability. If you and your partner need to make some major lifestyle decisions, being open and honest about how you feel is really important, as it could lead to an explosive and costly situation down the track. Maintaining regular social contacts is very

important for our health and well being, especially if you live alone, are widowed, or divorced.

6. **FUN**: If you are working on getting the right mix of the other five ingredients, this will be the icing on the cake! Variety is the spice of life. Create a mix of activities in your weekly planner, as mentioned in earlier sections. Live the width of your life, not just the length. Live in the present moment, not looking back at what was, or waiting for the future. There are many fun things you can do, that don't have to cost a lot of money.

The residents of an Over 50's Lifestyle Park in our town, range in age from late 50's to late 80's. A musical director moved there a couple of years ago and he instigated a musical production, ***"The Black and White Minstrel Show"*** which was a great success. A group of the residents of varying ages were in the production and they had a lot of fun putting it together. I went to see the show and it was fantastic. Speaking to some of the cast later, they said, that it gave such a lift to their spirits, being part of the production and being involved in something that gave them purpose, as well as being lots of fun. It was a new experience for many of the cast. One of the men said that it's important to have new experiences, to replace the one's that no longer were possible. He added that it's never too late to try new things. I can't wait to see the next production, which is in rehearsal as I write this.

Ask yourself – ***Would you rather be rich or live a rich life?***

I hope I have given you some insights on how to cook up that great life. Happy cooking!

REMEMBER TO......

- Bring harmony into your life.

- Assess your priorities.

- Let go of what is not important.

- Accept change and go with the flow.

- Nurture your body, mind and spirit.

- Change your thoughts, change your life.

- Enjoy your life NOW, while you can – It's never too late.

After the success of her first book, "So What Do We Do Now?" The Baby Boomers' Guide to Enjoying Retirement, Eva Bennett's second book, "As Time Goes By" Dealing With Life's Changes, explores the ways in which we can deal with the different kinds of major changes that can happen in our lives.

Eva shares the insights she has gained from many years of presenting at seminars, facilitating training programs and also the personal stories many people have shared with her. Her suggestions are clear, practical and easy to implement. They will help you deal with major life changes and make the most of the rest of your life.

Some of the areas covered include:-

- The 5 stages to move on from endings to new beginnings.
- Catch your thoughts and change your life.
- Slow down the ageing process.
- The 6 ingredients to cook up a great life.

www.plansretirement.com.au
email: eva.bennett@bigpond.com